A Doctor's Easy Guide to
GLP-1 for OBESITY
(Ozempic, Wegovy, Zepbound, Mounjaro etc)

Dr Prabhat Das
MD, PhD, FACP

Better Health with Dr Das Series

Disclaimer
This book is intended solely for educational and informational purposes. It is not meant to replace personal medical advice, diagnosis, or treatment. Although I am a licensed physician, reading this book does not establish a doctor–patient relationship. Each individual's health condition, medical history, and risk factors are unique. Any medical decision should be made in partnership with your own healthcare professional who understands your specific situation. Medical science is continually advancing. New research and updated guidelines may lead to changes in recommendations over time.

Paperback ISBN: 978-1-971672-06-9
eBook ISBN: 978-1-971672-07-6

Typeset in font *Garamond* by *Indica Infomedia*, New Delhi, India
Printed in the United States of America

About the Author

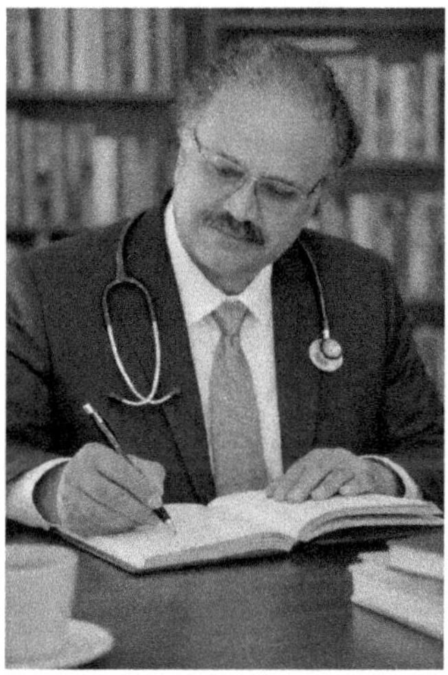

I am **Dr. Prabhat Das, MD, PhD, FACP**. My journey in medicine began in India, and for more than thirty five years I have had the privilege of practicing medicine in the United States. I trained in **Internal Medicine, Pulmonary Diseases, and Critical Care**, and throughout these decades medicine has been far more than a career for me. It has been a lifelong calling rooted in learning, service, and deep respect for the people who place their trust in their physician.

Over the course of my medical career, I have cared for patients in many different settings. I have seen patients in my office for everyday health concerns, treated people in busy emergency rooms, managed complex illnesses in the hospital, and cared for the most critically ill patients in intensive care units. Thousands of patients have sat across from me during office visits. Many more have depended on careful decisions made during difficult and urgent moments in the hospital and ICU.

But medicine is not only about diagnoses, tests, and treatments. Every day I have listened to patients speak about their worries, their fears, their uncertainty, and often the many questions they hesitate to ask. Those conversations have taught me something profound. People want clear information, honest guidance, and reassurance they can trust. They want to understand their health so they can take better care of themselves and the people they love.

These experiences have shaped how I think about health, illness, prevention, and the deeply human side of healing.

Through the **"Better Health with Dr Das" series**, I hope to reach many individuals I may never meet personally in my office. Many people struggle quietly with health questions and confusing medical information. My goal in these books is simple. I want to explain important medical topics in a clear, practical, and reassuring way so that readers feel informed, confident, and empowered to make better decisions about their health. The information presented in these books is based on reliable scientific knowledge and decades of clinical experience.

If these books bring clarity to someone who feels confused, comfort to someone who feels worried, or practical help to someone trying to improve their health, then this effort will have been deeply worthwhile.

Helping people live healthier, better informed lives continues to be one of the greatest privileges and satisfactions of my professional life.

Table of Contents

Introduction

Why I Wrote This Book

Over the years, one conversation has repeated itself again and again in my medical practice.

A patient sits across from me, often after years of struggling with weight. Sometimes they look discouraged. Sometimes they look embarrassed. And almost always they say something like this:

"Doctor, I have tried everything."

They describe diets that lasted a few weeks or a few months. They talk about exercise programs that started with enthusiasm but slowly faded. Some have tried commercial weight-loss programs, special foods, or strict meal plans. Many have experienced the same frustrating cycle: lose some weight, feel hopeful, and then gradually gain it back again.

After a while, people begin to blame themselves.

They think the problem must be a lack of discipline, a failure of willpower, or some personal weakness. This belief can quietly damage confidence and self-respect. I have seen many intelligent, hardworking people feel defeated by something they believe they should be able to control.

But over the years, medical science has taught us something important.

Weight regulation is far more complex than most of us once believed.

Our bodies are guided by powerful biological systems that influence hunger, fullness, metabolism, and energy balance. These systems involve hormones, the brain, the digestive tract, and many other organs working together. When these systems become disrupted, losing weight can become extremely difficult, even for people who are making genuine efforts.

This is why the conversation about obesity has begun to change.

Instead of seeing obesity only as a lifestyle problem, medicine increasingly recognizes it as a **chronic medical condition** that often requires a comprehensive approach to treatment.

Healthy eating and physical activity remain extremely important. But for many individuals, lifestyle changes alone are not always enough. Some patients need additional medical support.

That is where the story of **GLP-1 medicines** begins.

During the past decade, research into hormones that regulate appetite and metabolism has produced one of the most important advances in obesity treatment. Medications that mimic the hormone GLP-1 have shown the ability to reduce hunger, increase feelings of fullness, and support meaningful weight loss in many patients.

For the first time in many years, doctors have a treatment that works with the body's natural appetite-control system rather than simply trying to overpower it.

As news about these medications has spread, public interest has grown rapidly. Many people now hear about GLP-1 medicines through television programs, social media, or conversations with friends and coworkers.

Unfortunately, with rapid attention often comes confusion.

Some people believe these medicines are a miracle solution. Others believe they are dangerous or unnecessary. Many patients are unsure whom to trust or what information is accurate.

In my office, I began noticing that patients were arriving with many questions.

"Doctor, what exactly are these medicines?"

"Are they safe?"

"Will they really help me lose weight?"

"How long would I have to take them?"

"What happens if I stop?"

These are thoughtful and reasonable questions. They deserve careful answers.

That is the reason I decided to write this book.

My goal is not to promote any particular medication or create unrealistic expectations. Instead, my aim is to provide clear, balanced information so that readers can understand this new area of medicine.

In the chapters ahead, we will explore several important topics together. We will discuss what GLP-1 is and how it works in the body. We will look at how these medicines were developed and why they have attracted so much attention. We will also discuss who may benefit from these treatments, what side effects may occur, and what role lifestyle habits continue to play.

Just as important, we will talk about long-term health.

Weight loss alone is not the ultimate goal. The real objective is better overall health, improved energy, and a lower risk of serious conditions such as diabetes, heart disease, and fatty liver disease.

Throughout this book, I will try to explain the science in a way that is both accurate and understandable. Medical topics do not need to be confusing. With clear explanations, most people can understand the basic principles that influence their health.

I will also try to maintain a tone that I believe is very important in medicine: one that is calm, respectful, and free of judgment.

Struggles with weight are extremely common. Millions of people face this challenge, and many have done so for years. No one should feel ashamed for seeking help.

If this book accomplishes one important goal, I hope it helps replace frustration with understanding.

Knowledge allows people to make better decisions. It allows them to work more effectively with their doctors. And it often brings a sense of control that many people have been missing for a long time.

The story of GLP-1 medicines is still evolving. Research continues, and new discoveries are likely to appear in the years ahead. But even now, these treatments represent a meaningful step forward in our understanding of obesity and metabolic health.

This book is an invitation to explore that progress together.

By the time you reach the final chapter, my hope is that you will have a clear understanding of what GLP-1 medicines can do, what they cannot do, and how they may fit into a thoughtful plan for improving health.

Most importantly, I hope you will come away with a renewed sense of possibility.

Better health is rarely achieved overnight. It usually grows from steady, informed steps taken over time. And those steps can begin today.

Chapter 1

Obesity - Understanding the Real Problem

Obesity has become one of the most common health challenges of our time. In almost every country, and particularly in the United States, the number of people struggling with excess weight has steadily increased over the past several decades. Today millions of adults live with obesity, and many more are overweight and at risk of developing related health problems.

Yet despite how common this condition has become, obesity is still widely misunderstood.

Many people continue to think of obesity as a simple problem of eating too much and exercising too little. The solution, in this view, appears straightforward: eat less, move more, and the problem should disappear.

Unfortunately, real life is rarely that simple.

Anyone who has struggled with excess weight knows that losing weight is not always easy, even when a person is making sincere efforts. Many individuals follow diets, increase physical activity, and work hard to improve their habits. Some lose weight for a period of time, only to find that it slowly returns.

This cycle can be deeply frustrating.

Over time, people may begin to feel that they have failed in some personal way. They may believe that they simply lack the discipline or willpower required to succeed. This belief can quietly damage confidence and create unnecessary guilt.

Modern medical science tells us that this view is incomplete.

Obesity Is More Than a Cosmetic Issue

One of the most important things to understand about obesity is that it is not merely a matter of appearance. Excess weight can affect many organs and systems throughout the body.

Obesity increases the risk of several serious medical conditions, including:

- type 2 diabetes
- high blood pressure
- abnormal cholesterol levels
- heart disease and stroke
- fatty liver disease
- sleep apnea
- arthritis and joint problems

These conditions do not appear overnight. They often develop gradually over many years as excess weight places increasing stress on the body.

For this reason, doctors increasingly view obesity as a **chronic medical condition** rather than simply a lifestyle problem.

Recognizing obesity as a medical condition changes how we approach treatment. Instead of relying only on advice about dieting and exercise, doctors now consider a broader range of strategies that address the biological factors involved in weight regulation.

Why Weight Is So Difficult to Control

Human body weight is influenced by a complex system that involves the brain, hormones, metabolism, and the digestive system.

Deep inside the brain are centers that regulate hunger and fullness. These centers receive signals from many parts of the body. Hormones released from the stomach and intestines communicate information about recent meals. Fat tissue releases signals related to energy storage. Blood sugar levels also influence appetite.

Together, these signals help determine when we feel hungry and when we feel satisfied.

In an ideal situation, these systems maintain a balance between the calories we consume and the energy we use.

However, several factors can disrupt this balance.

Genetic influences may affect appetite and metabolism. Sleep deprivation can alter hunger hormones. Chronic stress can encourage overeating. Certain medications may also contribute to weight gain.

Modern food environments also play a role. Highly processed foods are widely available, convenient, and often designed to be extremely appealing. When these foods are combined with sedentary lifestyles, the biological systems that regulate appetite can become overwhelmed.

As a result, maintaining a healthy weight becomes much more difficult.

The Body's Resistance to Weight Loss

Another important concept in weight management is the body's tendency to resist weight loss.

When a person begins to lose weight, the body may respond by increasing hunger and reducing metabolic rate. In other words, the body attempts to conserve energy.

This response developed over thousands of years of human evolution. During ancient times, food shortages were common. The ability to regain lost weight quickly helped people survive periods of famine.

In today's world, however, these same protective mechanisms can make sustained weight loss challenging.

Many people experience this effect during dieting. At first weight may decrease steadily. But as time passes, hunger increases and progress slows. Eventually weight may begin to return.

Understanding this biological response helps explain why long-term weight management often requires more than simple calorie restriction.

A Changing View in Medicine

As scientific understanding has improved, doctors have begun to approach obesity in a new way.

Instead of focusing only on willpower and calorie counting, modern treatment strategies consider the hormonal and metabolic systems that regulate appetite and energy balance.

This shift has opened the door to new forms of treatment.

In addition to lifestyle changes, physicians now sometimes use medications that help regulate the biological signals involved in hunger and metabolism. These medications do not replace healthy habits, but they can support them by making appetite easier to manage.

One of the most important developments in this area involves a hormone called **GLP-1**.

Why New Treatments Are Needed

Traditional weight-loss advice remains valuable. Balanced nutrition, regular physical activity, adequate sleep, and stress management all play essential roles in maintaining health.

However, for some individuals these measures alone are not enough.

When biological signals strongly encourage hunger or reduce metabolic rate, maintaining long-term weight loss can become extremely difficult. Patients who repeatedly experience weight regain often feel discouraged.

New treatments aim to address these biological factors more directly.

GLP-1 medicines represent one of the most promising advances in this effort. By influencing appetite regulation and digestion, these medications help support the body's natural signals of fullness.

For many patients, this means that healthy eating habits become easier to maintain.

A New Chapter in Obesity Care

The growing interest in GLP-1 medicines reflects a broader change in the way doctors understand obesity.

Instead of blaming individuals for struggling with weight, medicine increasingly recognizes the complex biological forces involved. This understanding allows treatment to become more compassionate, more scientific, and more effective.

At the same time, it is important to maintain realistic expectations. No medication alone can solve the problem of obesity. Healthy habits remain essential for long-term success.

But when medical treatments and lifestyle changes work together, many people find that managing their weight becomes far more achievable.

Looking Ahead

In this chapter we have explored why obesity is more complicated than it may appear at first glance. Body weight is influenced by a network of biological signals involving the brain, hormones, metabolism, and the digestive system.

Recognizing these factors helps explain why weight loss can

be difficult and why new medical approaches have begun to emerge.

In the next chapter, we will focus on a key part of this system.

We will explore the hormone **GLP-1**, where it comes from, how it works in the body, and why it has become central to a new generation of treatments for obesity and metabolic disease.

Chapter 2

What Is GLP-1? The Hormone That Helps Control Hunger

To understand how modern medicines help with weight loss, we must first understand an important hormone that the body produces naturally. This hormone is called **GLP-1**, short for **glucagon-like peptide-1**.

Although the name sounds technical, the idea behind it is actually quite simple.

GLP-1 is one of the body's natural signals that helps regulate **hunger, digestion, and blood sugar after eating**. It is part of a complex communication system that allows the digestive system, pancreas, and brain to work together in maintaining energy balance.

Scientists did not originally study GLP-1 for weight loss. The hormone first attracted attention because of its role in **blood sugar control in people with diabetes**. Only later did researchers realize that it also had powerful effects on appetite and body weight.

Today, GLP-1 has become one of the most important hormones in modern obesity medicine.

The Body's Internal Communication System

Our bodies constantly send signals from one organ to another. These signals allow different systems to work together smoothly.

For example, when you eat a meal, several things happen almost immediately:

- Food enters the stomach and digestive process begins
- Nutrients move into the small intestine
- The pancreas prepares to release insulin
- The brain receives signals that food has been eaten

All of this coordination depends on hormones and nerve signals that communicate information throughout the body.

GLP-1 is one of the key hormones involved in this communication.

It acts as a messenger that informs the brain and pancreas that food has entered the digestive system.

Where GLP-1 Comes From

GLP-1 is produced by specialized cells located in the lining of the **small intestine**. These cells release the hormone shortly after food enters the digestive tract.

The release happens quickly. Within minutes of eating, GLP-1 levels in the bloodstream begin to rise.

Once released, the hormone travels through the bloodstream and affects several organs, including:

- the pancreas
- the stomach
- the brain

Through these actions, GLP-1 helps regulate digestion and appetite.

GLP-1 and Blood Sugar Control

One of the most important functions of GLP-1 is helping the body control blood sugar levels after meals.

When glucose from food enters the bloodstream, the pancreas releases insulin. Insulin allows glucose to move from the blood into the body's cells, where it can be used for energy.

GLP-1 supports this process in several ways.

First, it **stimulates the pancreas to release insulin** when blood sugar levels rise after eating.

Second, it **reduces the release of glucagon**, a hormone that causes the liver to release stored glucose into the bloodstream.

Together, these actions help prevent large spikes in blood sugar after meals.

Because of these effects, GLP-1 quickly became a focus of research in diabetes treatment.

Effects on the Brain and Appetite

As scientists studied GLP-1 more closely, they discovered that its influence was not limited to blood sugar.

The hormone also affects areas of the **brain that regulate hunger and satiety**.

When GLP-1 signals reach these brain centers, several changes occur:

- appetite decreases
- feelings of fullness increase
- cravings may become less intense

These signals help the body recognize that enough food has been consumed.

For individuals struggling with excess weight, this effect can make eating patterns easier to manage.

Slowing the Emptying of the Stomach

GLP-1 also affects how quickly food leaves the stomach.

Normally, after a meal, food gradually moves from the stomach into the small intestine. This process is called **gastric emptying**.

GLP-1 slows this process slightly. When the stomach empties more slowly:

- food remains in the stomach longer
- fullness lasts longer after meals

• hunger returns more gradually

This effect contributes to the appetite-regulating properties of GLP-1.

Why Natural GLP-1 Does Not Last Long

Although GLP-1 has important effects in the body, it naturally lasts only a short time.

An enzyme in the bloodstream quickly breaks down the hormone. Within a few minutes after being released, much of the GLP-1 has already been inactivated.

Because of this short lifespan, the hormone's effects are brief.

For many years, this rapid breakdown made it difficult to use GLP-1 directly as a medication. Scientists needed a way to reproduce its beneficial actions while allowing the effects to last much longer.

Eventually researchers succeeded in developing medications that mimic GLP-1 but remain active in the body for extended periods.

The Beginning of GLP-1 Medicines

Once scientists created longer-acting versions of GLP-1, a new class of medications emerged. These drugs are known as **GLP-1 receptor agonists**.

They work by activating the same receptors in the body that natural GLP-1 uses.

In other words, they imitate the actions of the body's own hormone, but their effects last much longer. Some remain active for an entire day, while others can work for a full week after a single injection.

Because these medicines enhance the body's natural appetite-control system, they help regulate hunger rather than simply suppress it.

This difference is one reason why they have attracted so much attention in recent years.

A Hormone with Multiple Benefits

GLP-1 is unique because it influences several aspects of metabolism at the same time.

Its actions include:

- stimulating insulin release
- reducing glucagon secretion
- slowing stomach emptying
- signaling fullness to the brain

Together, these effects support both **blood sugar control and appetite regulation**.

This combination makes GLP-1 an especially powerful target for medical treatments designed to address both diabetes and obesity.

Looking Ahead

Understanding GLP-1 helps explain why these medications have produced such promising results in clinical studies.

However, the journey from discovering a hormone in the intestine to developing modern medications took many years of scientific research.

In the next chapter, we will explore that story.

We will see how scientists discovered incretin hormones, how early experiments revealed the potential of GLP-1, and how decades of research eventually led to the medicines that are transforming the treatment of obesity and metabolic disease today.

Chapter 3

The Scientific Journey - From Discovery to Modern Medicine

Scientific discoveries rarely happen overnight. Most important medical advances develop slowly over many years, often through the work of many different researchers around the world.

The story of GLP-1 is a good example of this process.

Today GLP-1 medicines are widely discussed in connection with weight loss and diabetes treatment. But the journey that led to these medications began decades ago with a simple scientific observation about how the body responds to food.

An Interesting Observation About Glucose

Many years ago, scientists studying diabetes noticed something curious.

When people consumed glucose by mouth, their bodies released **much more insulin** than when the same amount of glucose was given directly into the bloodstream through an intravenous infusion.

This observation puzzled researchers. After all, glucose is the same molecule regardless of how it enters the body. Why should the body produce more insulin when glucose is eaten rather than injected?

Scientists suspected that the digestive system might be releasing signals that stimulate insulin production after meals.

This idea eventually led to the discovery of a group of hormones known as **incretins**.

The Incretin Effect

The term *incretin* refers to hormones released from the intestine that enhance insulin secretion after eating.

When food reaches the digestive tract, these hormones are released into the bloodstream and help the pancreas produce insulin. This mechanism helps the body control blood sugar after meals.

Two incretin hormones eventually became the focus of scientific research:

- **GIP (glucose-dependent insulinotropic polypeptide)**
- **GLP-1 (glucagon-like peptide-1)**

Both hormones play a role in regulating blood sugar, but GLP-1 soon attracted particular attention because it appeared to have additional effects on appetite and digestion.

Discovering GLP-1

GLP-1 was identified through studies of a larger molecule called **proglucagon**, which is produced in the pancreas and the intestine.

Researchers discovered that when proglucagon is processed in intestinal cells, it produces several smaller peptides. One of these peptides is GLP-1.

Further studies revealed that GLP-1 is released from specialized cells in the small intestine after food enters the digestive tract.

Once released, the hormone travels through the bloodstream and interacts with receptors located in several organs, including the pancreas, stomach, and brain.

Scientists soon realized that GLP-1 had several important actions:

- stimulating insulin release when blood sugar rises
- reducing the release of glucagon
- slowing stomach emptying
- influencing appetite and satiety

These effects made GLP-1 an attractive target for new treatments.

The Challenge of a Short-Lived Hormone

Although GLP-1 showed great promise, researchers quickly encountered an obstacle.

The natural hormone has an extremely **short lifespan in the bloodstream**. Within a few minutes after being released, it is broken down by an enzyme called **DPP-4 (dipeptidyl**

peptidase-4).

Because of this rapid breakdown, the hormone's effects disappear quickly.

This problem made it difficult to use GLP-1 directly as a medication. Any injected hormone would be destroyed almost immediately.

Scientists needed to find a way to create longer-lasting versions of GLP-1.

Developing GLP-1-Based Medicines

Researchers eventually solved this problem by developing molecules that mimic the action of GLP-1 but resist rapid breakdown in the bloodstream.

These medications are known as **GLP-1 receptor agonists**.

They activate the same receptors as natural GLP-1 but remain active in the body for much longer periods.

Some of the early medications required daily injections. Later developments produced longer-acting versions that could be given **once weekly**.

These improvements made treatment far more convenient for patients.

An Unexpected Discovery: Weight Loss

The first GLP-1 medications were developed primarily to treat **type 2 diabetes**. Their ability to stimulate insulin release and improve blood sugar control made them useful for managing this condition.

However, during clinical trials researchers noticed something unexpected.

Many patients taking these medications began to lose weight.

The weight loss was gradual but consistent. Participants reported reduced appetite and smaller portion sizes. They often felt full sooner during meals and less interested in snacking.

This observation opened a new area of research.

Scientists began studying whether GLP-1 medicines could be used specifically to treat **obesity**.

Expanding Research on Obesity Treatment

As clinical trials continued, the results became increasingly encouraging.

Studies showed that GLP-1–based medications could help many individuals achieve significant weight loss when combined with healthy lifestyle changes.

Patients often reported that the experience felt different from traditional dieting. Instead of constantly struggling with hunger, they felt more comfortable eating smaller meals.

This change in appetite regulation made long-term weight management easier for many people.

Over time, additional medications were developed that enhanced these effects even further.

A Rapidly Evolving Field

Today the field of metabolic medicine is evolving rapidly.

Researchers continue to study new medications that target the hormonal systems controlling appetite and metabolism. Some of these newer treatments combine the effects of GLP-1 with other hormones involved in energy balance.

These developments represent an important shift in the treatment of obesity.

Instead of relying solely on willpower and calorie restriction, modern therapies are beginning to address the biological systems that regulate hunger and metabolism.

Why This Scientific Story Matters

Understanding the history of GLP-1 helps explain why these medications have generated so much interest.

The development of these drugs was not an accidental discovery or a short-term trend. It represents decades of careful scientific work aimed at understanding how the body controls appetite and blood sugar.

This research has produced treatments that work with the body's natural systems rather than against them.

For many patients, that difference can make a significant impact on their ability to manage weight and improve overall health.

Looking Ahead

Now that we have explored the scientific journey behind GLP-1 medicines, the next step is to understand how these medications work inside the body in more detail.

Which organs do they affect?

How do they influence appetite and digestion?

Why do many patients feel satisfied with smaller meals?

In the next chapter, we will examine **the mechanism of action of GLP-1 medicines** and see how they interact with the brain, stomach, pancreas, and metabolism to support weight management.

Chapter 4

How GLP-1 Medicines Work Inside the Body

In the previous chapters we explored the discovery of GLP-1 and how scientists eventually developed medications that mimic its action. Now we can turn to a very practical question.

How do GLP-1 medicines actually work inside the body?

Understanding this helps explain why these medications can influence both blood sugar and body weight. The answer lies in the way GLP-1 interacts with several organs at the same time.

Rather than affecting a single part of the body, GLP-1 medicines influence multiple systems involved in appetite, digestion, and metabolism. The most important of these systems include:

- the brain
- the stomach
- the pancreas

• the liver and metabolism

Each of these effects contributes to the overall benefits seen during treatment.

The Brain: Regulating Hunger and Satiety

One of the most important actions of GLP-1 occurs in the brain.

Deep within the brain are centers that regulate appetite. These centers constantly receive signals from the body that indicate whether energy is needed or whether enough food has already been consumed.

When GLP-1 receptors in the brain are activated, several changes occur.

Appetite signals become less intense.

Feelings of fullness increase.

Food cravings may decrease.

As a result, many people feel satisfied with smaller portions than they previously required.

Patients often describe this experience in simple terms. They say that the constant thoughts about food become quieter. Eating becomes more controlled and less driven by hunger.

This change can make healthy eating habits much easier to maintain.

The Stomach: Slowing Gastric Emptying

GLP-1 medicines also influence how quickly food leaves the stomach.

Normally, after a meal, the stomach gradually empties its contents into the small intestine. This process, called **gastric emptying**, determines how long food remains in the stomach.

GLP-1 slows this process slightly.

When food remains in the stomach longer:

- the feeling of fullness lasts longer
- hunger returns more slowly
- meal portions often decrease naturally

Because of this effect, many patients notice that they feel satisfied sooner during meals.

The slowing of stomach emptying also contributes to better control of blood sugar after eating, because glucose enters the bloodstream more gradually.

The Pancreas: Supporting Insulin Release

Another key action of GLP-1 occurs in the pancreas.

After a meal, rising blood sugar levels signal the pancreas to release insulin. Insulin allows glucose to enter cells, where it can be used for energy.

GLP-1 enhances this process by stimulating insulin release when blood sugar levels are elevated.

At the same time, GLP-1 reduces the release of another hormone called **glucagon**. Glucagon normally tells the liver to release stored glucose into the bloodstream.

By reducing glucagon levels after meals, GLP-1 helps prevent excessive increases in blood sugar.

These combined actions make GLP-1 medicines particularly useful for individuals with type 2 diabetes.

Effects on the Liver and Metabolism

Although the brain, stomach, and pancreas receive the most attention, GLP-1 medicines also influence broader aspects of metabolism.

When appetite decreases and calorie intake becomes lower, the body begins to use stored energy from fat tissue. Gradually, body weight begins to decrease.

As weight loss occurs, several beneficial metabolic changes often follow.

These may include:

- improved insulin sensitivity
- lower blood pressure
- improved cholesterol levels
- reduction in fat accumulation in the liver

These improvements contribute to better overall metabolic health.

Why the Experience Feels Different from Dieting

Many patients say that weight loss during GLP-1 treatment feels different from previous attempts at dieting.

When people attempt strict calorie restriction without medical support, the body often reacts by increasing hunger signals. As a result, maintaining the diet becomes increasingly difficult.

GLP-1 medicines change this experience by influencing the biological signals that regulate appetite.

Instead of constantly fighting hunger, patients often feel that their body is cooperating with them.

This does not mean that healthy eating becomes unnecessary. Lifestyle habits remain extremely important. However, the medication can help create a biological environment that supports those habits.

A Combination of Effects

The benefits of GLP-1 therapy do not result from a single action. Instead, they arise from several effects occurring together.

The brain reduces appetite.

The stomach prolongs fullness.

The pancreas improves blood sugar control.

Metabolism gradually shifts toward a healthier balance.

Together, these actions create conditions that support steady weight loss and improved metabolic health.

HOW GLP-1 WORKS

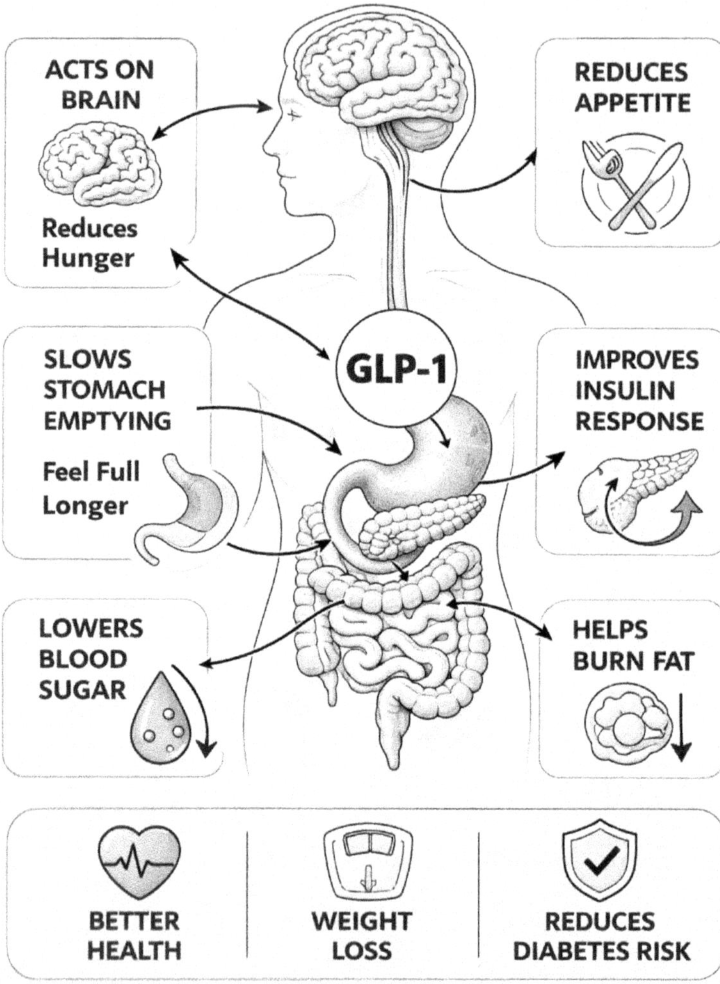

Looking Ahead

Now that we understand how GLP-1 medicines work in the body, the next important question becomes practical.

Who should consider these treatments, and who should not?

Not everyone with excess weight requires medication, and GLP-1 therapy is not appropriate for every individual.

In the next chapter we will explore the medical guidelines used by doctors to determine who may benefit from GLP-1 therapy and how these decisions are made in clinical practice.

Chapter 5

Who Can Benefit from GLP-1 Treatment?

After learning how GLP-1 medicines work inside the body, the next logical question is a practical one.

Who should consider using these medications?

Although GLP-1 therapy has received a great deal of public attention, it is not intended for everyone. Like any medical treatment, it must be used carefully and appropriately.

Doctors evaluate several factors before recommending these medications. The goal is to identify patients who are most likely to benefit while ensuring that treatment remains safe.

Understanding Body Mass Index

One of the first measurements doctors consider is **body mass index**, commonly called BMI.

BMI is a simple calculation based on a person's height and weight. It provides an estimate of body fat and helps classify weight into general categories.

The usual categories are:

- **BMI 18.5–24.9:** normal weight
- **BMI 25–29.9:** overweight
- **BMI 30 or higher:** obesity

Although BMI does not capture every aspect of body composition, it remains a useful starting point when evaluating weight-related health risks.

Medical guidelines commonly use BMI to determine when medication for weight management may be appropriate.

When Medication May Be Recommended

Doctors generally consider weight-loss medications in the following situations:

- **BMI of 30 or higher**, even without other medical problems
- **BMI of 27 or higher** when obesity-related conditions are present

These associated conditions may include:

- type 2 diabetes
- high blood pressure
- abnormal cholesterol levels
- fatty liver disease

• sleep apnea

• certain joint problems

In these situations, even moderate weight loss can improve health significantly. Medication may help patients achieve results that have been difficult to reach with lifestyle changes alone.

Patients with Type 2 Diabetes

GLP-1 medicines were originally developed for the treatment of type 2 diabetes. For patients who have both diabetes and excess weight, these medications may provide two important benefits.

They can help:

• improve blood sugar control

• support weight loss

Because excess weight often makes diabetes harder to manage, reducing weight can improve the effectiveness of other diabetes treatments.

In many cases, GLP-1 medicines are used alongside other diabetes medications as part of a comprehensive treatment plan.

When Lifestyle Changes Are Not Enough

Healthy lifestyle habits remain the foundation of weight management. Balanced nutrition, regular physical activity, adequate sleep, and stress management are essential for long-term health.

However, some individuals continue to struggle with weight despite making serious efforts to improve their habits.

Biological factors often play a role. Hormones that regulate appetite may remain strongly active. The body may resist weight loss by slowing metabolism or increasing hunger.

In these situations, medication may help correct some of these biological signals.

GLP-1 therapy works by supporting the body's natural appetite-regulation system, making it easier for many patients to maintain healthier eating patterns.

Patients with Cardiovascular Risk Factors

Excess weight contributes to several conditions that increase the risk of heart disease.

These include:

- high blood pressure
- elevated cholesterol levels
- insulin resistance
- inflammation

Weight reduction can improve many of these risk factors. For patients whose excess weight is contributing to cardiovascular risk, GLP-1 therapy may be considered as part of a broader plan to improve metabolic health.

The goal in these cases is not simply weight reduction for appearance. The objective is to reduce long-term health risks.

Who Should Not Use GLP-1 Medicines

Although GLP-1 therapy can be helpful for many patients, it is not suitable for everyone.

Doctors carefully evaluate medical history before prescribing these medications. Certain conditions may make their use inappropriate.

For example, individuals with a history of certain rare thyroid tumors or serious gastrointestinal disorders may need to avoid these medications.

Pregnancy is another important situation in which weight-loss medications are generally not recommended.

Because each patient's medical situation is unique, these decisions are best made with the guidance of a physician.

Setting Realistic Expectations

Another important aspect of starting GLP-1 therapy is understanding what the medication can and cannot do.

These medicines can help regulate appetite and support weight loss, but they are not a miracle cure.

Healthy eating habits, physical activity, and long-term lifestyle changes remain essential.

Patients who view medication as a **tool that supports healthy habits** usually achieve the best results.

Weight loss typically occurs gradually over several months rather than immediately.

A Shared Decision Between Patient and Doctor

The decision to begin GLP-1 therapy is usually made through a conversation between the patient and a healthcare professional.

During this discussion, the doctor may review:

- the patient's medical history
- previous weight-loss efforts
- current medications
- potential benefits and risks
- personal preferences

Together, the patient and doctor can decide whether this treatment fits into a comprehensive plan for improving health.

Looking Ahead

Now that we have discussed who may benefit from GLP-1 therapy, the next step is to examine the medications themselves.

Several drugs in this category are now available, and they differ in dosing schedules, strength, and convenience.

In the next chapter we will explore the **GLP-1 medicines currently available**, how they compare with one another, and how doctors help patients choose the most appropriate treatment.

Chapter 6

GLP-1 Medicines Available Today

Over the past decade, several medications based on the GLP-1 hormone have been developed. Although they work through similar biological mechanisms, they differ in their strength, dosing schedules, and the specific conditions they are used to treat.

Understanding these medications helps patients and physicians make informed decisions about treatment.

All of the medicines discussed in this chapter belong to a group called **GLP-1 receptor agonists**. This means they activate the same receptors in the body that natural GLP-1 uses. By doing so, they imitate the hormone's effects on appetite, digestion, and blood sugar control.

Some of these medications were first approved for diabetes treatment, while others were later approved specifically for obesity management.

Semaglutide

One of the most widely discussed medications in recent years is **semaglutide**.

Semaglutide belongs to the GLP-1 receptor agonist class and has been studied extensively in both diabetes and obesity treatment.

It is available in two commonly used forms:

• a formulation used primarily for diabetes

• a higher-dose formulation approved for chronic weight management

Semaglutide has a long duration of action, allowing it to be administered **once weekly**. The medication is given as a small injection under the skin.

Clinical studies have shown that semaglutide can help many patients achieve meaningful weight loss when combined with healthy lifestyle habits.

Tirzepatide

Another medication receiving significant attention is **tirzepatide**.

Although it is often discussed alongside GLP-1 medicines, tirzepatide is slightly different. It activates two hormone pathways involved in metabolic regulation:

• GLP-1 receptors

• GIP receptors

Because of this dual action, tirzepatide influences both appetite regulation and metabolic processes related to insulin and energy balance.

Like semaglutide, tirzepatide is administered as a **weekly injection** and has shown impressive results in studies involving weight reduction and blood sugar control.

Liraglutide

An earlier medication in the GLP-1 class is **liraglutide**.

Liraglutide was originally developed for diabetes treatment and later approved at a higher dose for chronic weight management.

Unlike semaglutide and tirzepatide, liraglutide is typically administered **once daily** rather than once weekly.

Although daily injections may seem less convenient, liraglutide remains an effective treatment for many patients and has a long track record of clinical use.

Dulaglutide and Related Medicines

Other GLP-1 receptor agonists have also been developed, including medications primarily used for diabetes management.

One example is **dulaglutide**, which is administered as a once-weekly injection. While its primary use is improving blood sugar control in patients with diabetes, it also tends to produce modest weight reduction.

Several other medications in this class share similar mechanisms and may be used depending on the patient's medical needs.

How These Medicines Are Taken

Most GLP-1 medicines are administered through **subcutaneous injections**, meaning they are injected just under the skin.

Common injection sites include:

- the abdomen
- the thigh
- the upper arm

The needles used for these injections are very small, and most patients find the process easier than they initially expected.

Many modern injection devices are designed as prefilled pens that simplify the process.

Some GLP-1 medications are taken **once weekly**, while others require **daily injections**.

An oral form of semaglutide is also available for diabetes treatment, although the injectable form is generally preferred for weight management.

Choosing the Right Medication

The choice of medication depends on several factors.

Doctors may consider:

- the patient's medical history
- whether diabetes is present
- the amount of weight loss needed

- convenience of dosing
- cost and insurance coverage
- potential side effects

In many cases, the decision becomes clear after discussing these factors with a physician.

Patients often prefer medications with weekly dosing because they are easier to incorporate into daily life. However, other factors may influence the final choice.

Individual Response Can Vary

It is important to remember that people do not all respond to medications in exactly the same way.

Some patients experience substantial weight loss, while others experience more modest changes.

Several factors may influence this response, including genetics, metabolism, lifestyle habits, and underlying medical conditions.

For this reason, treatment plans are often adjusted over time based on the patient's progress and tolerance of the medication.

Medication Is Only One Part of the Plan

Although GLP-1 medicines can play an important role in weight management, they work best when combined with healthy lifestyle habits.

Balanced nutrition, regular physical activity, adequate sleep, and stress management remain essential components of long-term health.

Medication helps regulate appetite and metabolism, but it does not replace the need for healthy daily habits.

Patients who combine medication with thoughtful lifestyle changes usually achieve the most sustainable results.

Looking Ahead

Now that we have reviewed the different GLP-1 medicines currently available, the next important topic is how treatment begins.

Doctors do not usually start patients at the highest dose immediately. Instead, treatment begins with a low dose that increases gradually over time.

In the next chapter, we will discuss **how GLP-1 therapy is started**, how doses are adjusted safely, and what patients can expect during the first few weeks of treatment.

Chapter 7

Starting GLP-1 Treatment – Doses and Titration

Once a patient and doctor decide that GLP-1 therapy may be appropriate, the next step is to begin treatment in a careful and controlled way. This stage is important because the body needs time to adjust to the medication.

Unlike many medications that start at a full dose immediately, GLP-1 medicines are usually introduced **gradually**. Doctors begin with a small dose and increase it slowly over several weeks.

This process is called **dose titration**.

Titration allows the body to adapt to the medication and helps reduce side effects, particularly those related to digestion.

Why Treatment Starts with a Low Dose

GLP-1 medicines influence several systems in the body,

including appetite regulation, stomach emptying, and blood sugar control. When these effects begin suddenly at a high dose, the body may react with uncomfortable symptoms.

Starting with a lower dose gives the digestive system time to adjust.

During the first few weeks, the medication begins to affect appetite and digestion gradually. Once the body becomes accustomed to the medication, the dose can be increased safely.

This gradual approach significantly improves comfort for most patients.

The Process of Dose Titration

Although the exact schedule varies depending on the medication used, the general pattern of treatment is similar.

Treatment usually progresses through three stages:

• **Initial phase** – a low starting dose for several weeks

• **Adjustment phase** – gradual dose increases at regular intervals

• **Maintenance phase** – the dose that provides the best balance between benefits and tolerability

Each step typically lasts several weeks, allowing the body to adjust before the next increase.

For many patients, it may take **two to three months** to reach the final maintenance dose.

Patience during this stage is very important.

What Patients Notice in the Early Weeks

During the first few weeks of treatment, patients may begin to notice subtle changes.

Common experiences include:

- feeling full sooner during meals
- reduced appetite
- less interest in snacking
- smaller portion sizes

These changes occur because the medication begins influencing the brain's hunger signals and slowing stomach emptying.

It is important to remember that weight loss may not occur immediately. The early phase of treatment focuses on allowing the body to adjust safely to the medication.

Gradual weight loss often begins once the medication reaches higher doses.

Learning the Injection Process

Most GLP-1 medications are administered by **subcutaneous injection**, meaning they are injected just beneath the skin.

Although the idea of injections may seem intimidating at first, the process is usually simple and nearly painless.

The needles used are extremely small, and the injection devices are designed to be easy to use.

Common injection sites include:

- the abdomen
- the thigh
- the upper arm

Healthcare professionals usually demonstrate the injection technique during the first visit. After a few attempts, most patients become comfortable performing the injection themselves.

Many medications are taken **once weekly**, which makes the routine easier to maintain.

Managing Mild Digestive Symptoms

Because GLP-1 medicines affect digestion, some patients experience mild gastrointestinal symptoms during the early weeks of treatment.

These symptoms may include:

- nausea
- mild stomach discomfort
- bloating
- constipation
- occasional diarrhea

In most cases, these effects are temporary and improve as the body adjusts to the medication.

Several practical steps can help minimize discomfort:

- eating smaller meals
- eating slowly

- avoiding very fatty or heavy foods
- stopping eating when comfortably full
- staying well hydrated

Following these habits allows the digestive system to adapt more comfortably.

Staying Consistent with Treatment

Consistency is important for GLP-1 therapy to work effectively.

Patients using weekly injections should try to take the medication on the **same day each week**. Establishing a routine helps ensure that doses are not forgotten.

Some people find it helpful to set reminders on their phone or calendar.

Maintaining a consistent schedule allows the medication to maintain steady levels in the body.

When to Contact Your Doctor

Although most patients tolerate GLP-1 medicines well, certain symptoms should prompt communication with a healthcare provider.

Patients should contact their doctor if they experience:

- severe or persistent nausea
- repeated vomiting
- intense abdominal pain

STARTING GLP-1

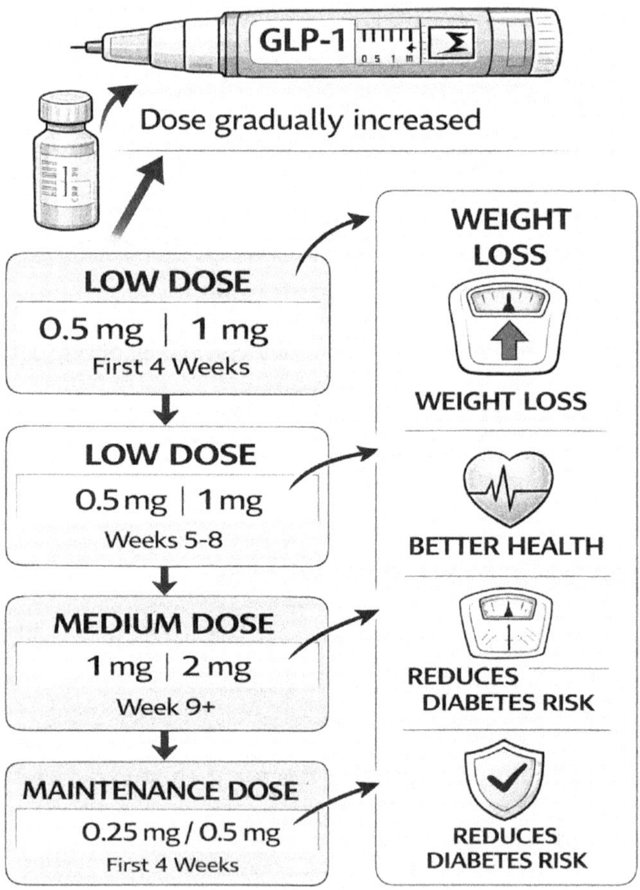

• symptoms of dehydration

• unusual weakness or dizziness

In many situations, adjusting the dose or slowing the titration schedule can resolve these problems.

Regular communication with a healthcare provider helps ensure safe and effective treatment.

The Importance of Patience

One of the most important things for patients beginning GLP-1 therapy to remember is that weight management takes time.

Rapid weight loss is rarely sustainable. The goal of treatment is steady, gradual improvement that can be maintained over the long term.

The titration process is designed to help patients reach an effective dose while minimizing discomfort.

With patience and consistency, the benefits of treatment often become clearer over the following months.

Looking Ahead

Once patients become comfortable with the medication and reach a stable dose, attention often shifts toward everyday habits that support long-term success.

In the next chapter, we will discuss **how to live successfully with GLP-1 therapy** and explore the daily habits that help patients achieve the greatest benefit from treatment.

Chapter 8

Living with GLP-1 Treatment - Daily Habits That Support Success

Beginning GLP-1 therapy is only the first step in the journey toward better health. Medication can help regulate appetite and metabolism, but the greatest benefits occur when treatment is combined with thoughtful daily habits.

Many patients discover that life with GLP-1 therapy feels different from previous attempts at dieting. Instead of constantly battling hunger, they often experience a calmer and more manageable relationship with food.

This change creates an opportunity to develop healthier patterns that can support long-term success.

Learning to Recognize New Hunger Signals

One of the first things many patients notice during treatment is that their appetite begins to change.

Meals that once seemed small may now feel satisfying. Hunger between meals may become less intense. Some people also notice that cravings for snacks gradually decrease.

Because of these changes, patients sometimes continue eating out of habit rather than hunger.

Learning to recognize the body's new signals becomes important.

Simple strategies can help:

• eat slowly and pause during meals

• notice when the feeling of fullness appears

• stop eating when comfortably satisfied rather than completely full

Over time, most people become more comfortable responding to these signals.

Adjusting Portion Sizes Naturally

GLP-1 medicines often make it easier to eat smaller portions without feeling deprived.

Rather than forcing strict restrictions, many doctors encourage patients to allow portion sizes to decrease naturally as appetite changes.

Balanced meals remain important. A healthy plate often includes:

• vegetables or fruits

• lean protein

- whole grains or other complex carbohydrates
- moderate amounts of healthy fats

This type of balanced nutrition helps maintain energy levels and supports overall metabolic health.

The Importance of Protein and Fiber

Two nutrients deserve special attention during weight management: **protein** and **fiber**.

Protein helps preserve muscle while weight is being lost. It also promotes satiety, helping people feel full after meals.

Fiber slows digestion and supports stable blood sugar levels. High-fiber foods also contribute to feelings of fullness.

Examples of protein-rich foods include:

- fish
- poultry
- eggs
- beans and lentils
- yogurt and cottage cheese

Examples of fiber-rich foods include:

- vegetables
- fruits
- whole grains
- legumes

- nuts and seeds

Including these foods regularly can strengthen the appetite-regulating effects of GLP-1 therapy.

Staying Well Hydrated

Adequate hydration is important for overall health and digestion.

Some patients experience mild constipation or digestive changes when beginning GLP-1 therapy. Drinking enough water throughout the day can help reduce these symptoms.

It is generally better to drink water regularly rather than waiting until thirst becomes noticeable.

Physical Activity Remains Essential

While GLP-1 medicines influence appetite, physical activity continues to play an important role in maintaining health.

Exercise offers several benefits:

- preserving muscle mass during weight loss
- improving cardiovascular health
- supporting metabolism
- improving mood and energy levels

The goal does not need to be intense exercise. Consistent movement is far more important than extreme effort.

Activities such as walking, cycling, swimming, or light strength training can all be beneficial.

Choosing activities that are enjoyable increases the likelihood that they will become part of a regular routine.

Sleep and Weight Regulation

Sleep is often overlooked in discussions about weight management, yet it plays a powerful role in metabolic health.

Poor sleep can disrupt hormones that regulate hunger and appetite. When sleep is inadequate, people may experience stronger cravings and reduced energy for physical activity.

Healthy sleep habits include:

- maintaining a regular sleep schedule
- limiting screen exposure before bedtime
- creating a comfortable sleep environment
- avoiding heavy meals late at night

Good sleep supports both physical health and emotional well-being.

Navigating Social Situations

Food plays an important role in social gatherings, celebrations, and family traditions. Many patients wonder how GLP-1 therapy will affect these situations.

In most cases, the experience becomes easier rather than more difficult.

Because appetite is better regulated, patients often find they can enjoy the same foods but in smaller portions.

Eating slowly and paying attention to fullness signals allows social meals to remain enjoyable without overeating.

Monitoring Progress

Weight management is rarely perfectly steady. Some weeks may show noticeable progress, while other weeks may show little change.

For this reason, doctors often recommend focusing on **long-term trends rather than daily fluctuations**.

Helpful ways to monitor progress include:

- weighing once a week
- noticing how clothing fits
- observing improvements in energy or physical activity
- tracking blood pressure or blood sugar when appropriate

These indicators often provide a better picture of health improvements than the scale alone.

Building Sustainable Habits

The ultimate goal of GLP-1 therapy is not simply weight loss. The real objective is building habits that support long-term health.

Medication can help regulate appetite, but lasting success depends on consistent daily choices.

Patients who combine treatment with balanced nutrition,

LIVING WITH GLP-1

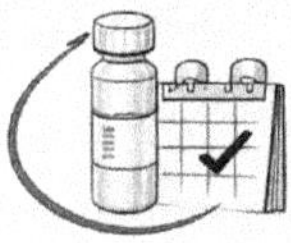

TAKE REGULAR INJECTIONS

Use as prescribed, inject regularly on schedule.

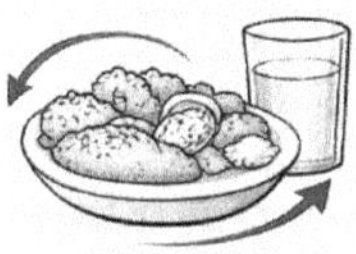

EAT HEALTHY & EXERCISE

Follow a balanced diet and increase physical activity.

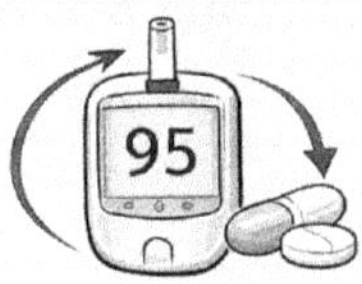

TRACK SUGAR & MEDS

Monitor blood sugar and take medications as directed.

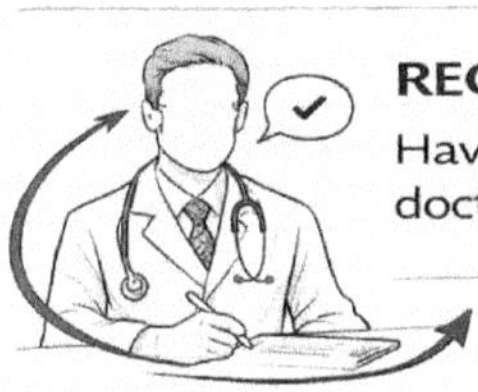

REGULAR CHECK-UPS

Have regular visits with your doctor to monitor progress.

BE PATIENT & AWARE

Weight loss takes time. Note any side effects & talk to your doctor.

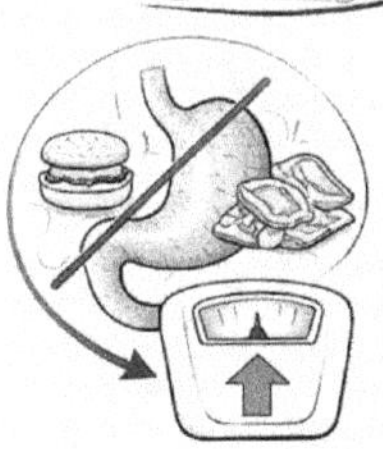

BE PATIENT & AWARE

Weight loss takes time. Note any side effects & talk to your doctor.

regular movement, adequate sleep, and stress management often achieve the most satisfying and sustainable results.

Looking Ahead

Although GLP-1 medicines offer many benefits, no medication is completely free of potential side effects.

Understanding these effects helps patients use the treatment safely and confidently.

In the next chapter, we will discuss **the most common side effects of GLP-1 therapy**, why they occur, and how patients can manage them effectively while continuing treatment.

Chapter 9

The Benefits of GLP-1 Therapy: More Than Just Weight Loss

When people hear about GLP-1 medicines, the first thing that usually comes to mind is weight loss. News reports, advertisements, and social media discussions often focus on the number of pounds that people lose while taking these medications.

Weight loss is certainly one of the most visible effects of GLP-1 therapy. However, the benefits of these medicines extend far beyond the number on the scale.

In clinical practice, doctors often see improvements in several aspects of metabolic health when patients use GLP-1 medications as part of a comprehensive treatment plan.

Understanding these broader benefits helps patients appreciate why these medicines have attracted so much attention in modern medicine.

Gradual and Meaningful Weight Loss

One of the most consistent effects observed with GLP-1 therapy is gradual weight reduction.

Weight loss usually occurs over several months rather than within a few weeks. This slower pace is often beneficial because gradual weight loss is more likely to be sustained over time.

Patients frequently report that eating smaller portions becomes easier because appetite signals are more manageable. Meals that once seemed small may now feel satisfying.

For many individuals, even a modest reduction in weight can produce meaningful improvements in health.

Studies have shown that losing **5 to 10 percent of body weight** can lead to improvements in blood pressure, blood sugar control, and cholesterol levels.

Improved Blood Sugar Control

GLP-1 medicines were originally developed to treat **type 2 diabetes**, and their ability to improve blood sugar control remains one of their most valuable benefits.

These medications help regulate blood glucose levels after meals by supporting insulin release and reducing the effects of glucagon.

For patients with diabetes, this can lead to several positive outcomes:

- lower average blood sugar levels
- improved HbA1c values

• fewer episodes of high blood sugar

Better blood sugar control can also lead to improved energy levels and reduced fatigue during daily activities.

Benefits for Heart Health

Excess weight often contributes to cardiovascular risk factors such as high blood pressure, abnormal cholesterol levels, and inflammation.

Weight reduction supported by GLP-1 therapy can help improve several of these factors.

Many patients experience:

• reductions in blood pressure

• improvements in cholesterol profiles

• improved metabolic health

These changes contribute to a healthier cardiovascular system and may reduce the long-term risk of heart disease.

Improvements in Fatty Liver Disease

Fat accumulation in the liver, often called **fatty liver disease**, has become increasingly common among individuals with obesity and metabolic syndrome.

Weight loss is one of the most effective strategies for improving this condition.

Because GLP-1 therapy often leads to gradual weight reduction and improved metabolism, many patients experience improvements in liver health over time.

Doctors sometimes monitor liver function tests during treatment to observe these changes.

Increased Energy and Physical Comfort

As weight decreases and metabolic health improves, many patients report noticeable changes in their daily lives.

These may include:

- increased energy
- improved mobility
- reduced joint discomfort
- greater ability to participate in physical activity

These improvements can create a positive cycle. Increased activity supports additional weight loss and further improvements in overall health.

Psychological and Emotional Benefits

Weight management can have a powerful influence on emotional well-being.

Many patients struggling with excess weight experience frustration, discouragement, or reduced self-confidence. When treatment begins to produce results, even modest ones, outlook and motivation often improve.

Patients may report:

- greater confidence
- improved mood
- reduced stress related to food and dieting

Some individuals also describe feeling relief from the constant mental focus on food that often accompanies strict dieting.

Looking Beyond the Scale

While weight reduction is important, doctors often encourage patients to evaluate progress using a broader perspective.

Positive changes may include:

- improved blood sugar control
- lower blood pressure
- healthier cholesterol levels
- increased energy
- better sleep quality

These improvements represent meaningful steps toward better long-term health.

A Tool for Long-Term Health

GLP-1 medicines are not intended to be quick fixes. Their greatest value lies in supporting long-term improvements in metabolic health.

BENEFITS OF GLP-1

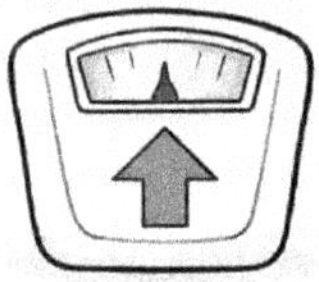

WEIGHT LOSS

Helps to reduce body weight through appetite and slowing digestion.

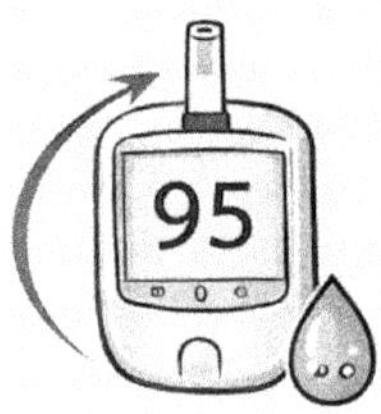

LOWERS BLOOD SUGAR

Improves blood sugar levels by increasing insulin release.

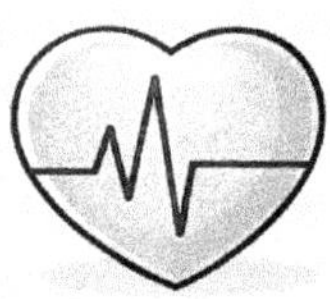

CARDIOVASCULAR HEALTH

May reduce the risk of heart attacks and strokes.

REDUCES DIABETES RISK

Helps to prevent or manage type 2 diabetes.

When combined with healthy lifestyle habits, these medications can help patients achieve sustainable progress toward better health.

Balanced nutrition, regular physical activity, adequate sleep, and stress management remain essential components of successful treatment.

Medication simply helps create a biological environment that makes these healthy habits easier to maintain.

Looking Ahead

Although GLP-1 therapy offers many benefits, it is important to understand that all medications can produce side effects.

Most side effects associated with GLP-1 medicines are mild and manageable, but patients should understand what to expect.

In the next chapter we will discuss **the potential side effects of GLP-1 medicines**, why they occur, and how they can be managed safely during treatment.

Chapter 10

Side Effects and Safety of GLP-1 Medicines

Whenever a new medication becomes widely used, two types of discussions often appear. Some people focus mainly on the benefits, while others concentrate on the risks. The truth, as is usually the case in medicine, lies somewhere between these two extremes.

GLP-1 medicines can provide important benefits for many individuals struggling with obesity or diabetes. At the same time, like all medications, they can produce side effects.

Understanding these effects allows patients to use the medication safely and with confidence. Fortunately, most side effects associated with GLP-1 therapy are **mild and temporary**, especially when treatment begins with a gradual increase in dose.

Why Side Effects Occur

Most of the side effects associated with GLP-1 medicines are related to the digestive system.

This should not be surprising. These medications influence appetite, slow stomach emptying, and affect how food moves through the digestive tract. When these changes occur, the digestive system may need time to adjust.

For many patients, mild symptoms appear during the early weeks of treatment and gradually improve as the body adapts.

The Most Common Side Effects

The most frequently reported side effects involve the gastrointestinal system.

These may include:

- nausea
- mild stomach discomfort
- bloating
- constipation
- occasional diarrhea

Among these, **nausea** is the most common.

Nausea usually occurs when treatment first begins or when the dose is increased. Because GLP-1 slows the emptying of the stomach, food may remain in the stomach longer than the body is accustomed to.

In most cases, this sensation improves after a few weeks.

Why Gradual Dose Increases Are Important

One of the most effective ways to reduce side effects is to increase the medication dose gradually.

Doctors typically start treatment with a low dose and increase it step by step over several weeks. This process allows the digestive system to adjust slowly.

Patients who follow this titration schedule often tolerate the medication very well.

Trying to increase the dose too quickly can increase the likelihood of nausea and other digestive symptoms.

Practical Ways to Reduce Digestive Symptoms

Several simple habits can help reduce digestive discomfort during GLP-1 treatment.

Patients often find relief by:

- eating smaller meals
- eating slowly
- avoiding very fatty or heavy foods
- stopping eating when comfortably full
- drinking adequate water

These strategies help the digestive system adapt to the medication more comfortably.

Many patients find that symptoms improve significantly within the first month of treatment.

Other Possible Side Effects

Although digestive symptoms are the most common, other mild side effects may occasionally occur.

These may include:

- headaches
- fatigue
- dizziness
- decreased appetite that feels stronger than expected

These symptoms are generally mild and tend to improve as the body adjusts to treatment.

If they persist, doctors may recommend adjusting the medication dose.

Gallbladder Issues

Rapid weight loss from any cause can increase the risk of gallstones. This effect is not unique to GLP-1 medicines; it can occur with many types of weight-loss treatments.

Symptoms of gallbladder problems may include:

- pain in the upper abdomen
- nausea after eating fatty meals

• pain that spreads toward the back or shoulder

Patients experiencing these symptoms should seek medical evaluation.

Pancreatitis

Inflammation of the pancreas, called **pancreatitis**, has been reported rarely in individuals using GLP-1 medicines.

Symptoms of pancreatitis may include:

• severe abdominal pain

• nausea and vomiting

• pain that worsens after eating

Although this complication is uncommon, patients experiencing severe abdominal pain should seek medical attention promptly.

Thyroid Considerations

Some GLP-1 medications carry warnings related to rare thyroid tumors observed in animal studies. Because of this, these medications are generally not recommended for individuals with certain rare types of thyroid cancer or related conditions.

Doctors review medical history carefully before prescribing these medications to ensure that treatment is appropriate.

Monitoring During Treatment

Regular follow-up visits help doctors ensure that GLP-1

therapy remains safe and effective.

During these visits, physicians may review:

- changes in weight
- possible side effects
- blood sugar levels
- overall health status

These evaluations allow the doctor to adjust treatment if necessary.

In many cases, minor adjustments in dosing can improve tolerance significantly.

Balancing Benefits and Risks

Every medical treatment requires balancing potential benefits against possible risks.

For individuals struggling with obesity or diabetes, the health risks associated with these conditions can be substantial. Excess weight increases the likelihood of heart disease, diabetes complications, joint problems, and several other conditions.

When GLP-1 medicines are used appropriately under medical supervision, the potential benefits often outweigh the risks for carefully selected patients.

Understanding both sides of the equation allows patients to make informed decisions about their treatment.

SIDE EFFECTS OF GLP-1

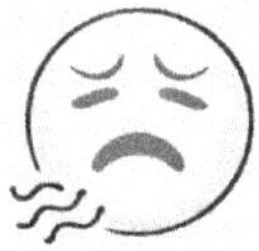

NAUSEA

Feeling queasy or like you might vomit.

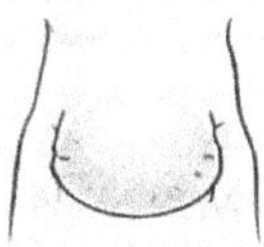

BLOATING

A full, swollen feeling in the stomach.

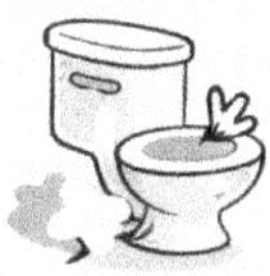

DIARRHEA

Frequent, loose, or watery stools.

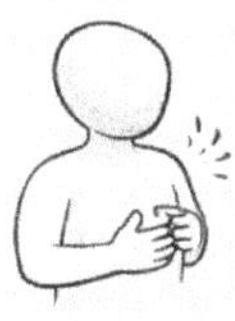

STOMACH PAIN

Cramping or discomfort in the abdomen.

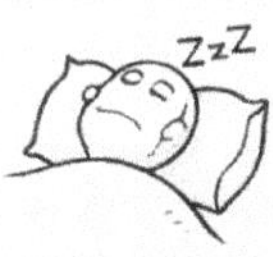

FATIGUE

Feeling tired or lacking energy.

Most side effects are mild and improve with time.

Looking Ahead

Now that we have discussed the safety and side effects of GLP-1 medicines, the next important topic is the role of medical supervision.

Why do doctors monitor patients carefully during treatment?

What tests may be recommended?

How do follow-up visits help maintain safety and effectiveness?

In the next chapter we will explore **why medical supervision is essential during GLP-1 therapy** and how regular follow-up helps ensure the best possible outcomes.

Chapter 11

Why Medical Supervision Is Essential During GLP-1 Treatment

The growing popularity of GLP-1 medicines has led many people to view them as simple weight-loss tools. News stories and social media discussions often focus on the dramatic results some individuals experience.

However, responsible medical care always involves more than simply taking a medication.

GLP-1 therapy works best when it is part of a thoughtful treatment plan guided by a healthcare professional. Medical supervision helps ensure that the treatment is safe, appropriate, and effective for each individual patient.

Just as doctors monitor patients taking medications for diabetes or high blood pressure, GLP-1 treatment also requires periodic evaluation and follow-up.

The Importance of a Careful Initial Evaluation

Before starting any weight-loss medication, physicians usually conduct a detailed medical evaluation.

This evaluation helps determine whether GLP-1 therapy is appropriate for the patient.

During this process, the doctor may review:

- medical history
- current medications
- previous attempts at weight loss
- family history of metabolic disease
- possible conditions that might affect treatment safety

A physical examination is usually performed as well. The doctor may measure weight, height, blood pressure, and other health indicators.

This initial assessment ensures that treatment decisions are based on a complete understanding of the patient's health.

Laboratory Tests Before Treatment

Doctors often recommend laboratory tests before beginning GLP-1 therapy.

These tests provide useful baseline information that helps guide treatment and allows future comparisons.

Common tests may include:

- blood glucose or HbA1c

- cholesterol levels
- liver function tests
- kidney function tests

By establishing baseline values, doctors can monitor how metabolic health changes during treatment.

Monitoring Progress During Treatment

Once treatment begins, regular follow-up visits help ensure that progress continues safely.

During these visits, physicians may evaluate:

- body weight
- appetite changes
- blood sugar levels
- blood pressure
- possible side effects

These visits also allow patients to discuss any concerns or questions about their treatment.

Monitoring progress helps doctors adjust the treatment plan when necessary.

Adjusting the Medication Dose

As discussed earlier, GLP-1 therapy usually begins with a low dose that gradually increases over time.

Medical supervision helps determine whether the dose should be increased, maintained, or occasionally reduced.

If side effects occur, the physician may slow the titration schedule or temporarily maintain a lower dose.

On the other hand, if the medication is well tolerated and weight loss has slowed, the doctor may recommend increasing the dose within the approved range.

This individualized approach helps maximize benefits while minimizing discomfort.

Reviewing Other Medications

Many patients who begin GLP-1 therapy are already taking medications for other conditions such as diabetes, high blood pressure, or high cholesterol.

As weight decreases and metabolic health improves, some of these medications may require adjustment.

For example:

• diabetes medications may need dose changes if blood sugar improves

• blood pressure medications may need adjustment if blood pressure decreases

These decisions should always be made under the guidance of a physician who understands the patient's overall treatment plan.

Monitoring Long-Term Health

One of the encouraging aspects of GLP-1 therapy is its potential to improve several markers of metabolic health.

As treatment continues, doctors may observe improvements in:

- blood sugar control
- blood pressure
- cholesterol levels
- body weight

Monitoring these changes allows physicians to assess the broader health benefits of treatment.

Communication Between Patient and Doctor

Successful treatment depends on open communication between patients and healthcare providers.

Patients should feel comfortable discussing their experiences with the medication, including both positive effects and challenges.

Important topics to discuss with a doctor may include:

- appetite changes
- digestive symptoms
- eating patterns
- weight changes

- emotional responses to treatment

These discussions help physicians tailor treatment to each patient's needs.

Avoiding Unsupervised Use

Because GLP-1 medicines have become widely discussed, some individuals attempt to obtain them without proper medical supervision.

This approach can be risky.

Without professional guidance, patients may not receive appropriate dosing instructions, may overlook important side effects, or may obtain medications that are not manufactured according to proper safety standards.

For these reasons, GLP-1 therapy should always be managed by a qualified healthcare professional.

Treatment as Part of a Long-Term Plan

Perhaps the most important role of medical supervision is placing GLP-1 therapy within a broader plan for long-term health.

Weight management is not a short-term project. It requires ongoing attention to lifestyle habits, metabolic health, and medical conditions.

Doctors help guide patients through this process, adjusting treatment when necessary and supporting healthy habits along the way.

WHY MEDICAL SUPERVISION IS NEEDED

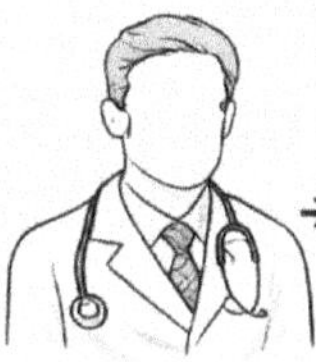

SAFE DOSE MANAGEMENT

→ Ensures the right dose is used and adjusted for you.

SIDE EFFECT MONITORING

→ Keeps a check on any adverse effects and manages them.

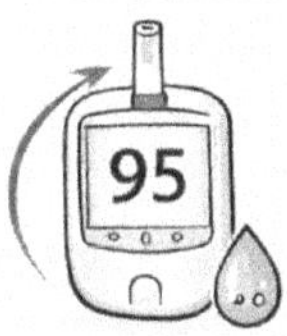

BLOOD SUGAR TRACKING

Monitors blood sugar levels to prevent insulin issues.

HEALTH PROTECTION

Reduces risks like heart problems and pancreatitis.

Doctors ensure safer and more effective treatment.

Looking Ahead

One of the most common questions patients ask about GLP-1 therapy concerns the duration of treatment.

How long should these medications be used?

Are they temporary tools, or do some patients need them for longer periods?

In the next chapter we will explore **how long GLP-1 treatment usually continues**, and how doctors decide whether ongoing therapy is appropriate.

Chapter 12

How Long Should GLP-1 Treatment Continue?

Sooner or later, almost every patient who begins GLP-1 therapy asks the same question:

How long will I need to take this medication?

This is a very reasonable concern. Many people hope that once they lose weight, they will be able to stop the medication and maintain their results permanently.

In some cases that may happen. However, in many situations the answer is more complex.

To understand why, we need to return to an important idea discussed earlier in this book: **obesity is often a chronic medical condition**. Like high blood pressure or diabetes, it may require long-term management rather than a short period of treatment.

The Body's Natural Response to Weight Loss

When a person begins to lose weight, several biological changes occur inside the body.

These changes may include:

- increased hunger signals
- reduced metabolic rate
- stronger cravings for calorie-dense foods

From an evolutionary perspective, these responses developed to protect the body during times when food was scarce. Regaining lost weight helped people survive.

In modern society, however, these same biological responses can make long-term weight management challenging.

Many individuals who lose weight through strict dieting eventually regain some or all of the lost weight because the body strongly encourages a return to its previous weight.

GLP-1 therapy helps counteract some of these signals by reducing appetite and supporting feelings of fullness.

Viewing Treatment as Long-Term Support

For some patients, GLP-1 therapy functions as **ongoing support for weight regulation**.

Instead of being used only for a few months, the medication may become part of a longer strategy for maintaining metabolic health.

This approach is similar to the way doctors manage other

chronic conditions. For example:

• blood pressure medications are often taken for many years

• cholesterol medications may continue long term

• diabetes treatments frequently require ongoing use

The goal is not simply short-term improvement but sustained health over time.

Individual Differences

Not every patient requires long-term medication.

Some individuals lose weight, adopt healthier habits, and maintain their progress after the medication is reduced or stopped.

Others find that appetite gradually increases again once treatment ends. In these situations, continuing medication may help preserve the progress that has already been achieved.

Doctors evaluate these situations individually.

Factors that influence the decision include:

• the amount of weight lost

• how stable the weight has remained

• the presence of diabetes or metabolic disease

• tolerance of the medication

• lifestyle habits and long-term goals

Together, the patient and physician decide whether continuing therapy is beneficial.

Periodic Reassessment

Even when GLP-1 therapy continues for an extended period, treatment should be reviewed regularly.

During follow-up visits, doctors may reassess:

- body weight and weight stability
- metabolic health markers
- possible side effects
- the patient's lifestyle habits
- long-term treatment goals

In some cases, the medication dose may be reduced after significant weight loss has been achieved.

In other cases, treatment may continue at a stable dose to maintain the benefits already gained.

Avoiding the Temporary-Fix Mindset

One of the common misunderstandings about weight-loss treatments is the expectation of a quick solution.

Many people have experienced cycles of strict dieting followed by weight regain. Because of these experiences, patients may hope that a new treatment will produce rapid results that permanently solve the problem.

In reality, long-term health improvements usually develop gradually.

GLP-1 therapy should be viewed as **a tool that supports long-**

term lifestyle change, not as a short-term shortcut.

Patients who approach treatment with patience and realistic expectations often achieve the most sustainable results.

The Role of Lifestyle Habits

Whether GLP-1 therapy continues for a few months or several years, healthy lifestyle habits remain essential.

Balanced nutrition, regular physical activity, adequate sleep, and stress management all support long-term weight stability.

Medication can help regulate appetite, but it works best when combined with these healthy habits.

Patients who focus on building sustainable routines often find that maintaining weight loss becomes easier over time.

An Ongoing Conversation

Because the duration of treatment varies from person to person, the question of how long to continue GLP-1 therapy should always be discussed with a healthcare professional.

Patients may wish to ask their doctor:

- What are my long-term treatment goals?
- How will we evaluate progress?
- When should we consider adjusting the dose?
- Under what circumstances might we stop treatment?

These discussions help ensure that the treatment plan remains appropriate and aligned with the patient's health goals.

Looking Ahead

Another important question naturally follows the discussion about treatment duration:

What happens if GLP-1 medication is stopped?

Some patients discontinue treatment after reaching their weight goals, while others may stop because of cost, side effects, or personal preference.

In the next chapter, we will explore **what typically happens after discontinuing GLP-1 therapy** and how patients can protect the progress they have achieved.

Chapter 13

What Happens After Stopping GLP-1 Treatment?

As patients progress through GLP-1 therapy and begin to see improvements in weight and metabolic health, an important question often arises:

What happens if the medication is stopped?

This is a thoughtful and practical concern. Many patients hope that once they lose weight, they will be able to discontinue the medication and maintain their progress without further treatment.

In some cases this is possible. However, in many situations the body's natural biology continues to influence appetite and weight regulation.

Understanding what may happen after stopping GLP-1 therapy can help patients prepare for the next stage of their health journey.

The Body's Weight Regulation System

Human body weight is controlled by a complex system involving the brain, hormones, metabolism, and digestive signals.

This system is designed to maintain stability. When body weight decreases significantly, the body often responds by activating mechanisms that encourage weight regain.

These mechanisms may include:

- increased hunger signals
- stronger cravings for calorie-dense foods
- reduced metabolic rate
- increased efficiency in storing energy

These responses developed during human evolution as protection against famine.

In modern life, however, they can make long-term weight maintenance difficult.

Appetite Changes After Discontinuation

One of the most noticeable changes after stopping GLP-1 therapy may involve appetite.

Because the medication helps regulate hunger signals, discontinuing it can allow those signals to return to their previous levels.

Some individuals notice that:

- hunger gradually increases
- feelings of fullness occur later during meals
- cravings for snacks become more frequent

These changes do not occur immediately for everyone, but they can develop gradually over time.

Recognizing these patterns early allows patients to respond with thoughtful lifestyle strategies.

Weight Regain in Some Individuals

Studies examining GLP-1 therapy have shown that some individuals regain part of the weight they lost after stopping treatment.

This does not mean that treatment was unsuccessful.

Even when some weight returns, patients often remain healthier than they were before treatment began. Blood sugar levels, blood pressure, and other metabolic markers may remain improved.

However, the possibility of partial weight regain is important to understand when planning long-term treatment.

Protecting the Progress Already Achieved

Although weight regain can occur, several strategies can help protect the progress achieved during treatment.

These strategies focus on maintaining the habits developed while taking the medication.

Helpful approaches may include:

- maintaining balanced eating patterns
- continuing regular physical activity
- monitoring weight periodically
- maintaining adequate sleep
- managing stress effectively

These habits strengthen the body's ability to maintain a healthier weight.

Gradual Discontinuation

In some situations, doctors may recommend reducing the medication dose gradually rather than stopping abruptly.

This gradual approach allows patients to observe how their appetite and weight respond as the medication decreases.

If appetite increases significantly or weight begins to rise rapidly, the treatment plan can be adjusted accordingly.

This strategy helps patients and physicians make informed decisions about long-term management.

When Continuing Treatment May Be Helpful

For some individuals, continuing GLP-1 therapy for a longer period may provide important benefits.

Patients who have experienced severe obesity, diabetes, or other metabolic conditions may find that ongoing treatment helps maintain both weight loss and metabolic health.

This decision should always be individualized.

Doctors consider several factors when recommending continued therapy, including:

- the patient's overall health
- the amount of weight lost
- the presence of diabetes or other conditions
- tolerance of the medication
- personal preferences and long-term goals

Shifting Focus to Lifestyle Foundations

Regardless of whether medication continues, the long-term success of weight management depends heavily on lifestyle habits.

Healthy eating patterns, physical activity, sleep, and stress management form the foundation of long-term metabolic health.

Patients who build strong routines during GLP-1 therapy often find it easier to maintain their progress even if medication is eventually discontinued.

The medication helps create an opportunity to develop these habits.

A Long-Term Perspective

Weight management is rarely a straight path. There may be periods of progress followed by periods of stabilization or minor setbacks.

The important point is that every step toward healthier habits and improved metabolic health contributes to long-term well-being.

Even when weight fluctuates, improvements in blood pressure, blood sugar, physical activity, and overall fitness remain valuable.

Patients should view their progress through this broader perspective.

Looking Ahead

As we approach the final chapter of this book, it is helpful to step back and consider the broader picture.

GLP-1 medicines represent an important medical advancement, but they are only one part of a larger strategy for achieving better health.

In the next chapter we will bring together the key ideas discussed throughout this book and explore **how patients can use GLP-1 therapy as part of a long-term plan for healthier living.**

Chapter 14

Using GLP-1 Therapy for Long-Term Health

Throughout this book we have explored many aspects of GLP-1 therapy. We have discussed how obesity develops, how the hormone GLP-1 works inside the body, how modern medications were developed, and how these medicines can help regulate appetite and support weight loss.

But knowledge alone is not enough.

The most important question for every reader is this:

How can this information be used in real life to improve health?

This final chapter brings together the key ideas discussed in earlier chapters and presents a practical roadmap for using GLP-1 therapy as part of a long-term strategy for better health.

Step One: Understanding the Real Nature of Obesity

The first step toward successful treatment is understanding that obesity is not simply a failure of willpower.

Modern research shows that body weight is influenced by many factors, including:

- appetite-regulating hormones
- brain signals that control hunger and satiety
- metabolism and energy balance
- sleep patterns and stress levels
- genetic influences

Recognizing this complexity allows patients to approach weight management with greater understanding and less self-blame.

GLP-1 therapy works by influencing some of these biological systems, helping restore balance in appetite regulation.

Step Two: Working with a Healthcare Professional

Weight management is most successful when patients work closely with a healthcare professional who understands their medical history and long-term health goals.

A doctor can help:

- determine whether GLP-1 therapy is appropriate
- choose the most suitable medication

• adjust doses safely

• monitor progress and side effects

Regular follow-up visits allow treatment to evolve as the patient's health improves.

Step Three: Building Healthy Eating Habits

Medication may reduce appetite, but food choices still play an essential role in overall health.

Balanced nutrition supports energy levels, muscle health, and metabolic stability.

Many patients benefit from focusing on:

• vegetables and fruits

• lean sources of protein

• whole grains

• healthy fats in moderate amounts

Eating slowly and paying attention to fullness signals often becomes easier during GLP-1 therapy.

This allows patients to develop a healthier relationship with food.

Step Four: Maintaining Regular Physical Activity

Physical activity remains one of the most powerful tools for improving health.

Exercise helps preserve muscle mass during weight loss and

supports cardiovascular health.

The goal does not need to be extreme or exhausting.

Many people achieve meaningful benefits through simple activities such as:

- daily walking
- cycling
- swimming
- light strength training

Consistency is more important than intensity.

Regular movement also improves mood, energy levels, and sleep quality.

Step Five: Protecting Sleep and Stress Balance

Sleep and stress have powerful effects on appetite and metabolism.

Poor sleep can increase hunger hormones and encourage overeating. Chronic stress can lead to emotional eating and disrupted metabolism.

Healthy routines that support good sleep and stress management may include:

- maintaining regular sleep hours
- limiting late-night screen exposure
- practicing relaxation techniques

• maintaining a balanced daily schedule

These habits strengthen the benefits of GLP-1 therapy.

Step Six: Monitoring Progress Realistically

Weight loss rarely occurs in a perfectly steady pattern.

Some weeks show noticeable changes, while other weeks may show little difference.

Patients benefit from focusing on long-term trends rather than short-term fluctuations.

Helpful indicators of progress include:

• gradual weight reduction

• improved blood pressure

• better blood sugar control

• increased physical stamina

• improved sleep and energy

These changes reflect meaningful improvements in health.

Step Seven: Planning for the Long Term

GLP-1 therapy may continue for months or, in some cases, years depending on individual circumstances.

Some patients eventually reduce or discontinue medication after reaching stable weight goals. Others may continue treatment longer to maintain the benefits they have achieved.

The key is developing habits that support long-term success.

Healthy routines built during treatment often remain valuable long after the medication is reduced or stopped.

A New Era in Obesity Care

The development of GLP-1 medicines represents an important milestone in the treatment of obesity and metabolic disease.

For many years, treatment options were limited. Patients often struggled with repeated cycles of dieting and weight regain.

Today, science has provided new tools that address the biological systems controlling hunger and metabolism.

These medications do not eliminate the need for healthy habits, but they can make those habits easier to maintain.

A Message of Encouragement

If you are struggling with excess weight, it is important to remember that you are not alone. Millions of people face similar challenges.

Weight management is not about perfection. It is about gradual progress and steady improvement.

Each healthy choice, each small change in daily habits, contributes to a healthier future.

GLP-1 therapy offers a new opportunity to support that journey.

Used thoughtfully, under medical guidance, and combined with healthy lifestyle habits, it can help many individuals

GLP-1 FOR LONG TERM HEALTH

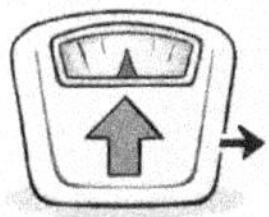

SUSTAINABLE WEIGHT LOSS

Supports gradual, maintainable weight loss.

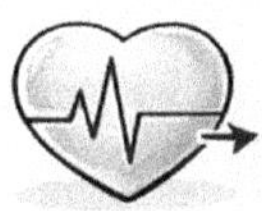

HEART HEALTH

May reduce the risk of heart disease and improve cardiovascular health.

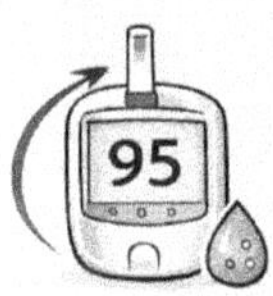

BETTER BLOOD SUGAR

Helps to control blood sugar levels and lower the risk of type 2 diabetes.

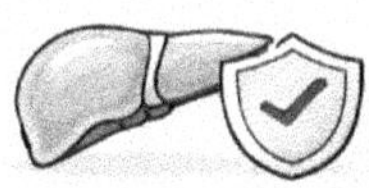

LIVER PROTECTION

Helps to reduce fat buildup in the liver and improve liver function.

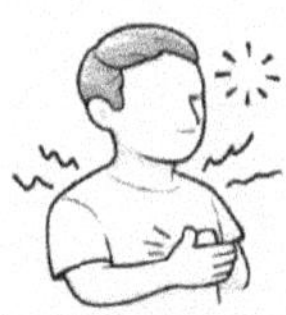

GLP-1 MEDICATIONS

Helps to control blood sugar levels and lower the risk of type 2 diabetes.

GLP-1 helps with lasting weight management and overall health improvement.

move toward better health, greater confidence, and a more active life.

And that, ultimately, is the true goal of every medical treatment.

Chapter 15

Frequently Asked Questions About GLP-1 Medicines

Over the past few years, GLP-1 medicines have attracted tremendous public attention. Patients often hear about them through television programs, news reports, social media discussions, or conversations with friends and family.

Because information often spreads quickly and sometimes without full context, many people are left with understandable questions. In my medical practice, patients frequently arrive with a mixture of curiosity, hope, and uncertainty.

This chapter addresses some of the most common questions about GLP-1 medicines in a clear and practical way. The goal is to help readers develop a balanced and realistic understanding of these medications.

What exactly are GLP-1 medicines?

GLP-1 medicines are medications that mimic the action of a natural hormone produced in the intestine called **glucagon-like peptide-1**, or GLP-1.

This hormone plays an important role in regulating several processes in the body after we eat. It helps stimulate insulin release, reduces the secretion of glucagon, slows the emptying of the stomach, and sends signals to the brain that promote feelings of fullness.

GLP-1 medications imitate these natural actions. By doing so, they help regulate appetite, improve blood sugar control, and support gradual weight loss.

Are GLP-1 medicines the same as insulin?

No. GLP-1 medicines and insulin are very different treatments.

Insulin directly lowers blood sugar by helping glucose enter the body's cells. People with diabetes may require insulin when their pancreas cannot produce enough of it.

GLP-1 medicines work indirectly. They encourage the pancreas to release insulin when blood sugar rises after meals. They also reduce appetite and slow stomach emptying.

Because of these additional effects, GLP-1 medicines can influence both blood sugar and body weight.

How much weight can people expect to lose?

Weight loss varies widely from person to person.

Clinical studies have shown that many individuals lose a meaningful amount of weight over time when GLP-1 medicines are combined with healthy lifestyle habits. In many studies, average weight loss ranges between **10 and 15 percent of body weight**, although some individuals lose more and others lose less.

The most important point is that weight loss usually occurs **gradually over several months** rather than quickly.

Even modest weight loss can produce important improvements in health, including better blood sugar control, lower blood pressure, and improved cholesterol levels.

How quickly do these medicines begin to work?

Some effects begin relatively early.

During the first few weeks of treatment, many patients notice that their appetite begins to decrease. They may feel satisfied with smaller portions and experience fewer cravings between meals.

However, noticeable weight loss usually takes time. As the medication dose increases gradually and eating habits adjust, weight reduction typically becomes more visible over several months.

Patience is important during this process.

Do I still need to watch my diet while taking these medicines?

Yes. GLP-1 medicines help regulate appetite, but they do not eliminate the need for healthy eating habits.

Balanced nutrition remains essential for maintaining overall health and supporting weight loss.

Many patients find that the medication makes it easier to adopt healthier eating patterns because hunger signals become less overwhelming.

Focusing on balanced meals that include vegetables, lean proteins, whole grains, and healthy fats can help maximize the benefits of treatment.

Do I still need to exercise?

Physical activity continues to play an important role in health and weight management.

Exercise helps maintain muscle mass during weight loss, supports cardiovascular health, and improves energy levels and mood.

The goal does not need to involve intense exercise. Consistent moderate activities such as walking, swimming, or cycling can provide substantial benefits.

Combining medication with regular movement produces the best results.

What happens if I miss a dose?

The exact recommendation depends on the medication being used.

For weekly injections, if a dose is missed and remembered within a few days, the patient may usually take the dose as soon as possible. If more time has passed, the next scheduled dose may simply be taken on the regular day.

Patients should always follow the specific instructions provided with their medication or consult their healthcare provider for guidance.

Maintaining a consistent schedule helps the medication work most effectively.

Are GLP-1 medicines addictive?

No. These medications are not addictive.

They do not stimulate the brain's reward systems in the way addictive substances do. Instead, they influence hormonal pathways that regulate appetite and digestion.

If the medication is discontinued, appetite signals may gradually return to their previous levels. This reflects the body's natural biology rather than addiction.

Can alcohol be consumed while taking GLP-1 medicines?

Moderate alcohol consumption may be acceptable for some individuals, but it should be discussed with a healthcare professional.

Alcohol contains calories and may affect blood sugar levels, particularly in patients with diabetes.

In addition, alcohol can sometimes worsen nausea or stomach discomfort when patients are beginning GLP-1 therapy.

Patients should use caution and follow their physician's guidance.

Are these medicines safe for older adults?

Many older adults can use GLP-1 medicines safely when treatment is carefully supervised by a physician.

Doctors consider several factors before prescribing these medications, including kidney function, other medical conditions, and current medications.

When used appropriately, GLP-1 therapy can sometimes provide meaningful benefits for older individuals struggling with obesity or diabetes.

Can GLP-1 medicines prevent diabetes?

Weight loss and improved metabolic health can significantly reduce the risk of developing type 2 diabetes in individuals with prediabetes.

Because GLP-1 medicines support weight reduction and improve blood sugar regulation, they may help lower the risk of progression to diabetes in some individuals.

However, medication alone is not sufficient. Healthy lifestyle habits remain the cornerstone of diabetes prevention.

Are these medicines appropriate for everyone who wants to lose weight?

No. GLP-1 medicines are generally prescribed for individuals with **obesity or overweight accompanied by weight-related medical conditions**.

Doctors evaluate each patient's health status carefully before recommending treatment.

This evaluation ensures that the potential benefits of the medication outweigh any possible risks.

A Final Word

Good medical care always begins with understanding.

Patients who ask questions and seek accurate information are better prepared to make thoughtful decisions about their health. GLP-1 medicines represent an important advance in the treatment of obesity and metabolic disease, but like all medical treatments they must be used wisely and under proper supervision.

When patients combine reliable information, medical guidance, and healthy daily habits, they place themselves in the best position to achieve lasting improvements in health.

Chapter 16
The Future of Obesity Treatment

Medicine is always evolving. New discoveries gradually change the way doctors understand disease and develop treatments. The story of GLP-1 medicines is part of a much larger scientific journey. What we are witnessing today is not the end of that journey, but the beginning of a new chapter in the treatment of obesity and metabolic disease.

For many years, obesity treatment relied mainly on lifestyle advice. Doctors encouraged patients to reduce calorie intake and increase physical activity. These recommendations remain essential and continue to form the foundation of good health. However, modern research has revealed that the biology of body weight is far more complex than previously understood.

Hormones, brain signals, metabolism, genetics, sleep patterns, and environmental factors all influence appetite and energy balance. As scientists continue to explore these systems, new treatment strategies are emerging that may further transform the management of obesity.

A New Scientific Understanding of Obesity

One of the most important changes in recent decades has been a shift in how obesity is viewed within the medical community.

In the past, obesity was often misunderstood as simply a failure of personal discipline. Patients frequently felt blamed for their weight struggles. This perception created frustration and discouraged many people from seeking medical help.

Modern science tells a very different story.

Research now shows that body weight is regulated by an intricate network involving the brain, the digestive system, fat tissue, and multiple hormones. These systems constantly communicate with each other to regulate hunger, fullness, and energy storage.

When these signals become disrupted, maintaining a healthy weight becomes extremely difficult, even for individuals who are making sincere efforts.

Recognizing obesity as a complex medical condition has opened the door to more effective and compassionate treatment strategies.

The Expanding Role of Hormone-Based Therapies

GLP-1 medicines represent one of the most important breakthroughs in this new approach. By mimicking the action of a natural hormone involved in appetite regulation, these medications help restore balance to the body's hunger signals.

The success of GLP-1 therapy has encouraged scientists to explore other hormones involved in energy regulation.

Researchers have discovered that the body uses several hormonal pathways to regulate appetite and metabolism. These include hormones that influence satiety, insulin release, fat metabolism, and energy expenditure.

Future treatments may combine the effects of multiple hormones in order to achieve stronger and more sustained results.

Dual and Triple Hormone Therapies

One of the most promising developments in this field involves medications that activate more than one hormonal pathway at the same time.

Some newer treatments already combine the effects of GLP-1 with another hormone called **GIP**, which also plays a role in insulin secretion and metabolic regulation.

Researchers are now investigating therapies that may influence **three hormonal pathways simultaneously**. These medications attempt to reproduce the complex biological signals that normally regulate appetite and energy balance in the human body.

Early research suggests that these multi-hormone therapies may produce substantial weight reduction while also improving blood sugar control and metabolic health.

Although research is still ongoing, these developments illustrate how rapidly the field is advancing.

Benefits Beyond Weight Loss

Another important area of research focuses on the broader health effects of these medications.

Excess weight is associated with several serious health conditions, including heart disease, type 2 diabetes, fatty liver disease, and certain forms of kidney disease.

Researchers are studying whether hormone-based therapies such as GLP-1 medicines may help improve these conditions directly, beyond their effects on weight loss.

Clinical studies have already shown encouraging results in some areas, particularly in reducing cardiovascular risk factors in patients with diabetes.

As more long-term studies become available, doctors will gain a clearer understanding of how these medications influence overall health.

The Promise of Personalized Medicine

Another exciting development in modern medicine is the concept of **personalized treatment**.

Not all patients respond to medications in the same way. Some individuals lose weight rapidly, while others experience more gradual changes. Genetic factors, metabolism, lifestyle habits, and medical conditions all influence these responses.

In the future, doctors may be able to tailor obesity treatments more precisely based on a patient's individual biology.

Advances in genetic research and metabolic testing may allow physicians to select the most effective treatment strategy for each person.

This approach could improve results and reduce unnecessary trial-and-error in treatment decisions.

Integrating Technology with Medical Treatment

Technology is also beginning to play a larger role in weight management.

Mobile health applications, wearable devices, and digital health platforms can help patients monitor their physical activity, sleep patterns, and nutritional habits.

These tools can provide valuable feedback and help patients maintain motivation during long-term treatment.

In the future, digital health systems may become more closely integrated with medical care. Doctors may be able to track certain health indicators remotely and adjust treatment plans based on real-time information.

This integration of technology and medicine may help improve long-term outcomes.

The Continuing Importance of Lifestyle

Despite the excitement surrounding new medications and scientific advances, one principle remains unchanged.

Healthy lifestyle habits will always be the foundation of long-term health.

Balanced nutrition, regular physical activity, adequate sleep, and stress management remain essential for maintaining metabolic health. No medication can completely replace these habits.

Instead, modern treatments should be viewed as tools that support healthier behaviors.

GLP-1 medicines and future therapies can help regulate appetite and metabolism, making it easier for patients to adopt and maintain healthier lifestyles.

A Future of Hope and Progress

The rapid development of new obesity treatments reflects a growing recognition that this condition deserves the same scientific attention as other major medical problems.

Researchers, physicians, and public health experts are now working together to better understand the biological systems that regulate body weight.

Each new discovery brings us closer to more effective and compassionate approaches to treatment.

For patients who have struggled with weight for many years, this progress offers a message of hope.

Modern medicine is beginning to provide tools that address the biological factors involved in obesity rather than relying solely on willpower and calorie restriction.

When these scientific advances are combined with healthy daily habits and supportive medical care, they create new possibilities for improving health and quality of life.

The future of obesity treatment is still unfolding, but it is clearly moving toward a more informed, more compassionate, and more effective approach to helping people live healthier lives.

Appendix A

Sample Meal Structure for Patients Using GLP-1

When patients begin GLP-1 therapy, one of the most common questions they ask is, "What should I eat now?"

Many people expect that they must follow a complicated or highly restrictive diet. In reality, the goal is usually much simpler. The most effective approach is to adopt **balanced, consistent, and sustainable eating habits** that work well with the appetite-regulating effects of GLP-1 medicines.

Because these medications often reduce hunger and increase the feeling of fullness, many patients naturally begin eating smaller portions. This creates an opportunity to develop healthier meal patterns that support long-term weight control and metabolic health.

This appendix provides a practical meal structure that patients can use as a guide.

A Simple Daily Eating Pattern

Most individuals do well with **three balanced meals and one optional small snack** during the day.

The goal is to maintain steady energy levels while avoiding large fluctuations in hunger.

A typical daily structure might look like this:

Time	Meal
Morning	Breakfast
Midday	Lunch
Afternoon (optional)	Light snack
Evening	Dinner

Because GLP-1 medicines slow stomach emptying and increase fullness, many patients find that they no longer need frequent snacks between meals.

The Balanced Plate Approach

One of the easiest ways to build healthy meals is the **balanced plate method**.

Imagine dividing your plate into sections:

Portion of Plate	Food Type
Half of the plate	Vegetables or fruits
One quarter	Lean protein
One quarter	Whole grains or complex carbohydrates

A small amount of healthy fat can also be included.

This structure helps maintain balanced nutrition while controlling calorie intake.

The Importance of Protein

Protein plays an especially important role during weight loss.

When people lose weight, the body may lose some muscle along with fat. Adequate protein intake helps protect muscle mass and supports metabolism.

Good sources of protein include:

- fish
- chicken or turkey
- eggs
- beans and lentils
- tofu
- yogurt or cottage cheese
- nuts and seeds

Including protein at each meal helps maintain fullness and supports steady energy levels.

The Role of Fiber

Fiber is another important component of healthy eating, particularly for individuals using GLP-1 medicines.

Fiber slows digestion, stabilizes blood sugar levels, and helps maintain a feeling of fullness.

Foods rich in fiber include:

- vegetables
- fruits
- whole grains
- legumes
- nuts and seeds

High-fiber foods also support digestive health and may help reduce constipation, which can occasionally occur during GLP-1 therapy.

Example Breakfast Options

Because GLP-1 medicines reduce appetite, breakfast does not need to be large. A balanced meal that includes protein and fiber is usually sufficient.

Examples include:

- Greek yogurt with berries and a small handful of nuts
- oatmeal with fruit and a spoonful of peanut butter
- eggs with whole-grain toast and vegetables
- cottage cheese with sliced fruit
- a smoothie made with yogurt, fruit, and protein powder

The goal is to start the day with steady energy rather than a heavy meal.

Example Lunch Options

Lunch should provide balanced nutrition and help sustain energy during the afternoon.

Examples include:

• grilled chicken salad with mixed vegetables and olive oil dressing

• vegetable soup with beans or lentils and whole-grain bread

• tuna or salmon salad with leafy greens

• brown rice with vegetables and grilled tofu or chicken

• a whole-grain sandwich with lean protein and vegetables

Eating slowly and paying attention to fullness signals is especially important.

Example Dinner Options

Dinner is often the largest meal of the day, but patients taking GLP-1 medicines frequently find that smaller portions feel more comfortable.

Balanced dinner ideas include:

• grilled fish with roasted vegetables and quinoa

• baked chicken with sweet potatoes and green beans

• stir-fried vegetables with tofu or shrimp and brown rice

- lentil curry with vegetables
- vegetable pasta with grilled chicken

Stopping when comfortably full helps prevent digestive discomfort.

Healthy Snack Ideas

Some individuals may not need snacks while using GLP-1 therapy, but a light snack can be helpful if hunger appears between meals.

Examples include:

- a small apple with peanut butter
- a handful of nuts
- yogurt
- carrot sticks with hummus
- a piece of fruit with cottage cheese

Snacks should be simple and moderate in portion size.

Eating Habits That Work Well with GLP-1 Therapy

Because these medicines slow stomach emptying and influence digestion, certain habits can improve comfort.

Helpful practices include:

- eating slowly

DIET DURING GLP-1 TREATMENT

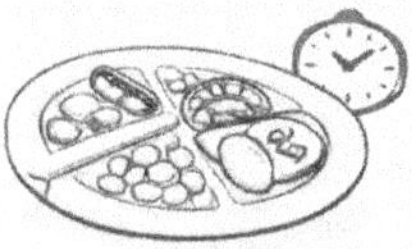

SMALL, FREQUENT MEALS

Eat smaller, regular meals throughout the day.

LIMIT UNHEALTHY FOODS

Cut back on high-fat, high-sugar, and processed foods.

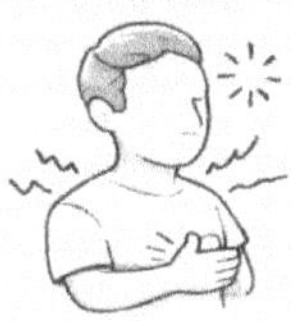

EAT SLOWLY

Chew thoroughly and take your time while eating.

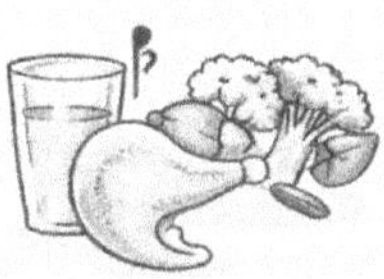

FOCUS ON PROTEIN & VEGGIES

Prioritize lean protein and vegetables in your meals.

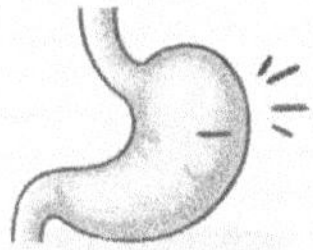

AVOID OVEREATING

Stop eating when you feel satisfed or full.

A healthy diet supports GLP-1 treatment and weight loss.

- choosing smaller portions
- avoiding very heavy or greasy meals
- stopping when comfortably full
- drinking water regularly

These habits help the digestive system adjust to the medication.

A Flexible Approach

There is no single diet that works for everyone. Cultural preferences, family traditions, and personal tastes all influence food choices.

The goal of this meal structure is not strict restriction but **balanced and sustainable eating habits**.

Patients who focus on simple, nutritious meals and pay attention to hunger and fullness signals often find that healthy eating becomes easier during GLP-1 therapy.

Combined with regular physical activity and medical supervision, these habits can support lasting improvements in weight and overall health.

Appendix B
A Simple Physical Activity Plan

When people begin treatment with GLP-1 medicines, much of the attention naturally focuses on changes in appetite and eating habits. However, physical activity remains an essential part of long-term health and weight management.

Exercise supports weight loss, protects muscle mass, improves cardiovascular health, and enhances overall well-being. Many patients also notice improvements in mood, energy levels, and sleep when they begin moving more regularly.

The goal of this appendix is not to prescribe a demanding exercise program. Instead, it offers a **simple and practical plan** that most people can begin safely and gradually.

Why Physical Activity Matters

Weight loss through medication and dietary changes often leads to a reduction in both fat and muscle mass. Maintaining muscle is important because muscle tissue supports metabolism and helps the body use energy more efficiently.

Regular physical activity helps:

- preserve muscle during weight loss
- improve heart and lung function
- support healthy blood pressure
- improve blood sugar control
- strengthen bones and joints
- improve mood and mental health

These benefits make physical activity an essential companion to GLP-1 therapy.

Start Slowly and Build Gradually

One of the most common mistakes people make when beginning an exercise program is trying to do too much too quickly.

A better strategy is to start gently and increase activity gradually. This approach reduces the risk of injury and makes the routine easier to maintain.

For many individuals, **walking** is the ideal starting point.

Walking requires no special equipment, places minimal stress on joints, and can be adjusted easily to match individual fitness levels.

A Simple Walking Program

The following four-week walking plan can help beginners develop a consistent routine.

Week	Activity Goal
Week 1	Walk 10–15 minutes per day, 5 days per week
Week 2	Walk 15–20 minutes per day, 5 days per week
Week 3	Walk 20–25 minutes per day, 5 days per week
Week 4	Walk 25–30 minutes per day, 5 days per week

After several weeks, many individuals feel comfortable walking **30 minutes most days of the week**. This level of activity provides meaningful health benefits.

Patients who enjoy walking may gradually increase either the distance or the pace.

Adding Strength Training

While walking supports cardiovascular health, strength training helps maintain muscle mass during weight loss.

Strength exercises do not require a gym membership. Many simple exercises can be performed at home using body weight or light resistance.

Examples include:

- chair squats
- wall push-ups
- light dumbbell exercises

• resistance band exercises

A simple routine performed **two to three times per week** can help strengthen major muscle groups.

For beginners, performing one or two sets of each exercise is usually sufficient.

Stretching and Flexibility

Stretching helps maintain flexibility and reduces muscle stiffness.

Gentle stretching after walking or exercise can improve comfort and mobility.

Examples include:

• calf stretches

• hamstring stretches

• shoulder stretches

• gentle back stretches

Stretching should be performed slowly without forcing the muscles.

Holding each stretch for about **15 to 20 seconds** is usually sufficient.

Incorporating Movement Into Daily Life

Not all physical activity needs to occur during structured exercise sessions. Daily habits also play an important role.

Simple ways to increase movement include:

- taking the stairs when possible
- parking slightly farther from entrances
- walking during phone calls
- doing light household tasks
- gardening or yard work

These small changes gradually increase daily energy expenditure.

Listening to the Body

When beginning any new activity program, it is important to listen to the body's signals.

Mild muscle soreness may occur during the early stages of exercise, but pain or discomfort that persists should be evaluated.

Patients should stop exercising and consult their physician if they experience:

- chest pain
- severe shortness of breath
- dizziness
- joint pain that worsens with activity

Most individuals can exercise safely, but medical guidance is important when underlying health conditions are present.

PHYSICAL ACTIVITY DURING GLP-1 THERAPY

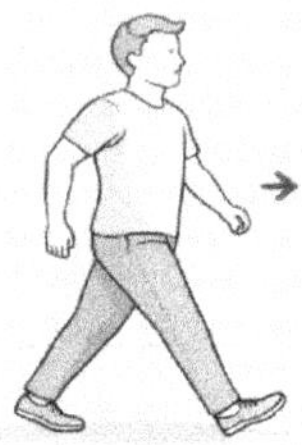

REGULAR EXERCISE

→ Be active most days, aiming for 150 min/week.

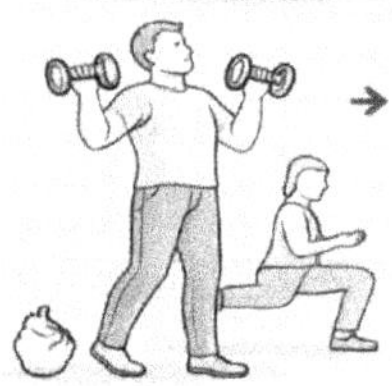

MIX IT UP

→ Combine aerobic, strength, & flexibility exercises.

START SLOWLY

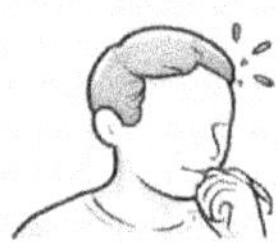

→ Begin at a comfortable pace and gradually increase.

MOVE MORE

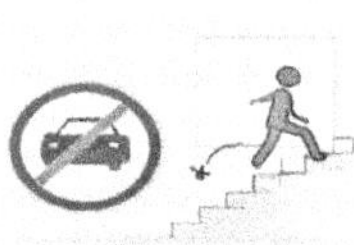

Choose to walk, take the stairs, or park farther away.

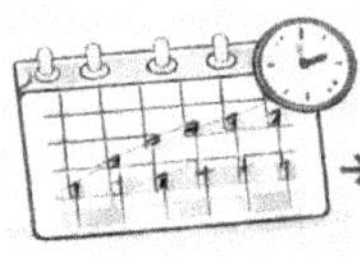

MAKE IT A HABIT

→ Find physical activities you like and stick with them.

Regular activity during GLP-1 therapy improves weight loss and overall health.

Staying Consistent

The greatest benefits of physical activity come from **consistency rather than intensity**.

Short periods of activity performed regularly are far more effective than occasional strenuous workouts.

Many people find that scheduling activity at the same time each day helps establish a routine.

Walking with a friend, listening to music, or exercising outdoors can also make physical activity more enjoyable.

A Long-Term Investment in Health

Physical activity is not merely a tool for weight loss. It is one of the most powerful habits for protecting long-term health.

Regular movement improves heart health, strengthens muscles and bones, supports metabolism, and contributes to emotional well-being.

When combined with balanced nutrition, adequate sleep, and appropriate medical care, physical activity becomes a cornerstone of healthy living.

For patients using GLP-1 therapy, developing a consistent movement routine greatly enhances the long-term benefits of treatment.

Appendix C
Monitoring Your Progress

When people begin a program to improve their health, it is natural to focus mainly on the number on the scale. While body weight is an important indicator, it is only one part of the larger picture.

Successful health improvement involves many changes that occur gradually over time. Blood pressure may improve, blood sugar may become better controlled, physical endurance may increase, and daily energy levels may rise.

Monitoring progress helps patients stay motivated and allows both patients and doctors to understand how treatment is working. This appendix provides a simple and practical approach to tracking these changes.

Why Monitoring Matters

Progress in health and weight management rarely occurs in a perfectly steady pattern. Some weeks may show noticeable improvement, while other weeks may show little change.

Without regular monitoring, it can be difficult to recognize gradual improvements that are taking place.

Tracking progress can help patients:

- recognize positive changes early
- stay motivated during slow periods
- identify habits that support success
- share useful information with their healthcare provider

Monitoring does not need to be complicated. A few simple measurements can provide valuable insight.

Tracking Body Weight

Body weight remains one of the most visible indicators of progress.

However, daily weight measurements can sometimes be misleading. Weight naturally fluctuates from day to day due to factors such as hydration, salt intake, and digestion.

For most people, weighing **once a week** at the same time of day provides a clearer picture of long-term trends.

Helpful tips include:

- weigh on the same day each week
- weigh at the same time of day
- use the same scale

• record the measurement consistently

The goal is to observe gradual trends rather than short-term fluctuations.

Measuring Waist Circumference

Waist circumference is another useful measurement.

Excess fat around the abdomen is closely linked with metabolic conditions such as diabetes and heart disease. As weight loss occurs, the waist measurement often decreases as well.

To measure waist circumference:

1. Stand upright and relax the abdomen.

2. Place the measuring tape around the waist at the level of the navel.

3. Record the measurement without pulling the tape too tightly.

Measuring once every two to four weeks is usually sufficient.

Monitoring Blood Pressure

For patients with high blood pressure or cardiovascular risk factors, monitoring blood pressure can provide important information.

Home blood pressure monitors are widely available and easy to use.

Recording blood pressure once or twice per week can help patients observe improvements that often accompany weight loss and healthier habits.

Patients should share these measurements with their healthcare provider during follow-up visits.

Monitoring Blood Sugar

Individuals with diabetes or prediabetes may benefit from monitoring blood sugar levels.

GLP-1 medicines often improve blood sugar control, and observing these changes can be encouraging.

Depending on medical advice, patients may monitor:

- fasting blood sugar
- blood sugar after meals
- HbA1c levels during routine medical visits

These measurements help doctors evaluate the effectiveness of treatment.

Observing Changes in Energy and Physical Ability

Not all improvements can be measured with numbers.

Many patients notice important changes in their daily lives as their health improves. These changes may include:

- increased energy
- improved stamina during walking or exercise

- better sleep quality
- reduced joint discomfort
- improved mood

Recording these observations can provide powerful motivation to continue healthy habits.

A Simple Progress Tracking Table

Keeping a written record of progress can be very helpful. The following table provides a simple way to track several key indicators.

Week	Weight	Waist Measurement	Blood Pressure	Notes
Week 1				
Week 2				
Week 3				
Week 4				
Week 5				
Week 6				

The notes column can be used to record observations such as exercise activity, changes in appetite, or other health improvements.

Avoiding Discouragement

It is important to remember that progress is rarely perfectly steady.

Some weeks may show little change in weight, even when healthy habits are being followed. This does not mean that the effort is unsuccessful.

Many health improvements occur gradually and may not immediately appear on the scale.

Focusing on long-term trends rather than short-term fluctuations helps maintain perspective and motivation.

Sharing Progress With Your Doctor

Regular monitoring also helps support productive conversations with healthcare providers.

When patients bring their records to medical appointments, doctors can review trends and adjust treatment plans if necessary.

This collaborative approach helps ensure that treatment remains safe and effective.

A Tool for Long-Term Success

Monitoring progress is not meant to create pressure or anxiety. Instead, it should serve as a simple tool that supports awareness and motivation.

Small improvements, repeated consistently over time, can

MONITORING THE PROGRESS DURING GLP-1

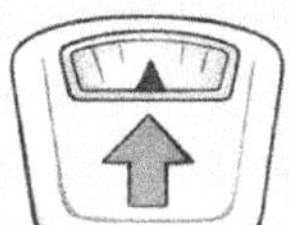

TRACK WEIGHT LOSS

→ Weigh yourself regularly to monitor weight changes.

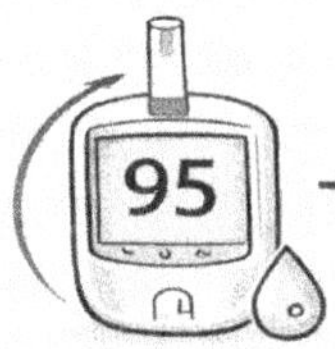

CHECK BLOOD SUGAR

→ Measure your blood sugar levels as directed by your doctor,

RECORD FOOD & ACTIVITY

→ Keep a record of meals, physical activity, and any symptoms.

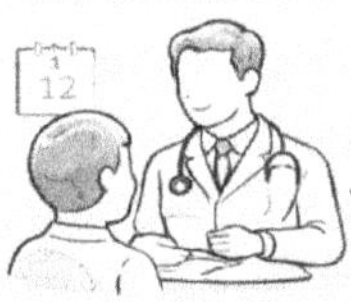

SEE YOUR DOCTOR

→ Have regular appointments for ongoing assessment.

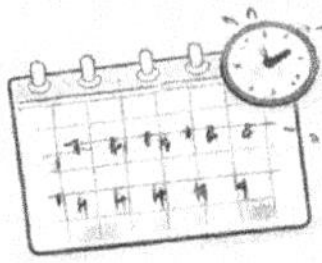

MAKE IT A HABIT

→ Find physical activittes you like and stick with them.

Tracking helps ensure safe and effective treatment

produce remarkable changes in health.

When patients observe these improvements, they often gain confidence and motivation to continue the journey toward better health.

With thoughtful monitoring, steady habits, and proper medical guidance, long-term health improvement becomes an achievable and rewarding goal

Thank You and Please Review the Book

Thank you for taking the time to read this book. I sincerely hope it has helped you understand your health a little more clearly and has given you practical, everyday steps you can follow with confidence. If you found this book helpful, **I would truly appreciate it if you could leave a brief and honest review.** Even a few lines sharing your experience can make a meaningful difference. Your feedback helps other readers find reliable, trustworthy health information and supports them in making better decisions for themselves and their families.

Warm regards,

Dr Prabhat Das

Continue your Healthcare Journey

Good health is a journey, not a single step. It is not achieved in one day or with one book. That is why I created the "Better Health with Dr Das" series, with each book addressing a different common condition. If you would like easy, practical guidance on other everyday health concerns, you may wish to explore the rest of books in this series.

Books in this series:

- A Doctor's Easy Guide to Understanding & Managing **OBESITY**.
- A Doctor's Easy Guide to Understanding & Managing **HIGH BLOOD PRESSURE**.
- Doctor, What **DIET** Is Best for Me?
- A Doctor's Easy Guide to **GLP-1 for OBESITY** (Ozempic, Wegovy, Zepbound, Mounjaro etc)
- Doctor, Why Can't I **Lose Weight?** A Doctor's Simple Guide to Safe & Sustainable Weight Loss

www.ingramcontent.com/pod-product-compliance
Ingram Content Group UK Ltd.
Pitfield, Milton Keynes, MK11 3LW, UK
UKHW021959270726
14060UKWH00003B/592